W9-ADJ-223

Quick Medical Terminology

A Self-Teaching Guide

5th Edition

Shirley Soltesz Steiner, R.N., M.S.

Natalie Pate Capps, M.N.Sc., R.N.

John Wiley & Sons, Inc.

This book is printed on acid-free paper ♾

Copyright © 2003 by Shirley Steiner. Copyright © 2011 by Shirley Steiner and Natalie Capps. All rights reserved

Published by John Wiley & Sons, Inc., Hoboken, New Jersey
Published simultaneously in Canada

No part of this publication may be reproduced, stored in a retrieval system, or transmitted in any form or by any means, electronic, mechanical, photocopying, recording, scanning, or otherwise, except as permitted under Section 107 or 108 of the 1976 United States Copyright Act, without either the prior written permission of the Publisher, or authorization through payment of the appropriate per-copy fee to the Copyright Clearance Center, 222 Rosewood Drive, Danvers, MA 01923, (978) 750-8400, fax (978) 646-8600, or on the web at www.copyright.com. Requests to the Publisher for permission should be addressed to the Permissions Department, John Wiley & Sons, Inc., 111 River Street, Hoboken, NJ 07030, (201) 748-6011, fax (201) 748-6008, or online at http:/www.wiley.com/go/permissions.

Limit of Liability/Disclaimer of Warranty: While the publisher and the author have used their best efforts in preparing this book, they make no representations or warranties with respect to the accuracy or completeness of the contents of this book and specifically disclaim any implied warranties of merchantability or fitness for a particular purpose. No warranty may be created or extended by sales representatives or written sales materials. The advice and strategies contained herein may not be suitable for your situation. You should consult with a professional where appropriate. Neither the publisher nor the author shall be liable for any loss of profit or any other commercial damages, including but not limited to special, incidental, consequential, or other damages.

For general information about our other products and services, please contact our Customer Care Department within the United States at (800) 762-2974, outside the United States at (317) 572-3993 or fax (317) 572-4002.

Wiley also publishes its books in a variety of electronic formats and by print-on-demand. Some content that appears in standard print versions of this book may not be available in other formats. For more information about Wiley products, visit our website at www.wiley.com.

ISBN 978-0-470-88619-9 (paper); ISBN 978-1-118-06373-6 (ebk);
ISBN 978-1-118-06374-3 (ebk); ISBN 978-1-118-06375-0 (ebk)

Printed in the United States of America

10 9 8 7 6 5

For

Dorothy Elizabeth Wilson Soltesz, who is my mom and best friend.

Mildred Hall, who is my godmother and may not know how much she influenced my growing-up years. Mildred assured me I had what it takes to go to college, get an education, and create a better life.

—S. S.

For

My perfect mate, Barry, and remarkable children, Harden, Pate, and Jacqueline Capps

My parents and sisters, who shaped me:
Susie Ashworth, Nick Pate, Amy Bean, and Molly Pate

With affection, gratitude, and adoration for you all.

—N. C.

Contents

To the Reader

What This Book Is and Who It's For

So you want to learn the language of medicine. Great! Everything you need for learning medical terminology is right in your hands. The language of medicine is precise and technically oriented. It is among the great tools of the mind for better understanding and more accurate communication between all practitioners of the life sciences. Learning this special language is your opportunity to be among them. *Quick Medical Terminology* can prepare you for a new job or even a new career in one of the nation's fastest growing job markets, health care and allied health services.

In *Quick Medical Terminology* you'll learn to pronounce, spell, and define medical terms used in today's health care settings. You will use a word-building strategy that helps you discover connections and relationships among word roots, prefixes, and suffixes. You'll learn the meaning of each part of a complex medical term and be able to put the parts together and define the term. Very quickly you'll develop a large repertoire of useful medical terms, much greater than the 500-plus terms presented in this text.

Beginning with Chapter 4, most of the medical terms in each chapter will focus on a particular part of the body. Grouping related terms in this way will help you learn them better. However, the order of the chapters should not be confused with the order of a standard head-to-toe medical evaluation. At the end of the book, there is a Review by Body System Assessment that will walk you through the standard head-to-toe examination medical professionals typically follow. This review will bring together the medical terminology you will learn in the rest of the book.

Quick Medical Terminology is an enjoyable way to learn the very special language of medicine by yourself, at your own pace. If you speak and understand English and have a high school education or equivalent, you'll quickly learn the basics and much more.

How to Use This Program

We suggest you use the following steps to approach your learning.

Step 1. Pre- and Post-Testing

If it's worth learning, isn't it worth knowing you have succeeded? You will find two Final Self-Tests in the back of your guide. We suggest you take one test before you begin your study and take another after you have completed all your lessons. Pre- and post-testing shows you how much you have learned. Either one of the final tests may be used first.

Step 2. Self-Instructional Chapter

This self-teaching guide lets you proceed at a pace that is right for you. It provides everything you need to complete each of the eleven instructional chapters, which include:

Introduction and Mini-Glossary. The first page of each chapter introduces you to what you will cover and provides a Mini-Glossary of the terms and word parts you'll be learning. You may want to refer to it as you proceed through the lesson.

Numbered frames. Numbered frames are the building blocks of each chapter. A frame presents a small amount of information and expects you to read and think about that information. Then it asks you to respond to it.

The way you respond may be:

- to select a medical term or definition from a list of suggested answers.
- to write a medical term for a given definition.
- to draw a conclusion and write it in your own words.

Example
Emesis is a term that means vomiting. A term that means excessive vomiting is *hyperemesis.* Underline the part of the medical term meaning excessive.

A gallbladder attack can cause excessive vomiting. Write the term that describes this unpleasant condition. ________________

Example
Myelo / dysplasia means defective development of the spinal cord.

Chondro means cartilage. What does chondro / dysplasia mean? ________________

Answers. As you work through the chapter, you'll find the correct answers on the left-hand side of the page. It's a good idea to use a folded piece of paper to cover the answer until you give your own. Your answer will be correct most of the time, but when your answer doesn't match ours, be sure you know why it doesn't. You may need to go back and review a few frames before continuing.

Pronunciation Guide. When you work with a medical term for the first time, the answer column guides your pronunciation of the new term. Take the opportunity to practice pronouncing each new term correctly several times. Say it aloud or subverbally (saying it to yourself).

Example
chondrodysplasia (kon′dro dis pla′zhe)

Review Exercises. Some chapters are longer than others, so to help you plan your breaks, we designed several short learning sequences into each chapter. A brief Review Exercise occurs at the end of a learning sequence. If you need a break, stop after a Review Exercise. Proceed at a pace that is right for you. We urge you to complete an entire chapter before calling it a day.

Summary Exercise. Each of the eleven instructional chapters ends with a Summary Exercise. This final exercise pulls together all the new terms you worked with in the chapter. Using the pronunciation guide alongside each term in the list, take the opportunity to practice pronouncing each term correctly and defining it aloud or subverbally. It really works! You might ask a friend to pronounce each term in the list so you can practice spelling it when you hear it.
[This is a good classroom exercise for instructor-guided spelling practice, pronunciation practice, and defining the terms.]

Chapter Self-Test. Each chapter ends with a Self-Test in two parts. Part 1 asks you to match a list of definitions with the correct medical terms. Part 2 asks you to construct the correct medical term for each definition listed. All terms and definitions are covered in the instructional chapter you have just completed. Here's another opportunity to see how you're doing.

Step 3. Chapter Review Sheet

Beginning on page 261, you'll find a two-part Review Sheet for each of the eleven chapters of instruction that make up this self-teaching program. We suggest you begin every new chapter (beginning with Chapter 2) by completing a Review Sheet for the previous chapter. These exercises are an important part of the learning program and will help you recall and practice the terms and definitions of the preceding chapter before you begin the next one.

Part 1: Given a term, or word part, write the meaning.

Part 2: Given the definition of a term, write the correct term.

Correct answers are provided.

You may use these Review Sheets anytime, and as often as you wish. We suggest you make several photocopies of each Review Sheet and use them at any time to practice what you've already covered. There is never enough practice.

Objectives of the Program

When you have finished *Quick Medical Terminology,* you will have formed well over 500 medical terms using our word-building strategy combining prefixes, suffixes, and word roots to create complex medical terms.

1. You will learn to understand medical terms by breaking them into their component parts and learning the meaning of the parts.
2. You will learn to construct medical terms from component parts to express given definitions.
3. You will learn to pronounce, spell, and define medical terms used in this book.
4. You will be able to apply this word-building strategy to terms covered in this book and other terms you will come across as you work in a health care setting.

Pronunciation Key

The primary stress mark (′) is placed after the syllable bearing the heavier stress or accent; the secondary stress mark (′) follows a syllable having a somewhat lighter stress, as in *com·men·da·tion* (kom′ ən·dā′ shən).

a	add, map	m	move, seem	u	up, done
ā	ace, rate	n	nice, tin	er	urn, term
air	care, air	ng	ring, song	yo͞o	use, few
ä	palm, father	o	odd, hot	v	vain, eve
b	bat, rub	ō	open, so	w	win, away
ch	check, catch	ô	order, jaw	y	yet, yearn
d	dog, rod	oi	oil, boy	z	zest, muse
e	end, pet	ou	out, now	zh	vision, pleasure
ē	even, tree	o͞o	pool, food	ə	the schwa, an
f	fit, half	oo	took, full		unstressed vowel
g	go, log	p	pit, stop		representing the
h	hope, hate	r	run, poor		sound spelled
i	it, give	s	see, pass		*a* in *above*
ī	ice, write	sh	sure, rush		*e* in *sicken*
j	joy, ledge	t	talk, sit		*i* in *clarity*
k	cool, take	th	thin, both		*o* in *melon*
l	look, rule	th	this, bathe		*u* in *focus*

Source: Slightly modified "Pronunciation Key" in *Funk & Wagnalls Standard College Dictionary*. Copyright © 1977 by Harper & Row, Publishers, Inc. Reprinted by permission of the publisher.

The schwa (ə) varies widely in quality from a sound close to the (u) in *up* to a sound close to the (i) in *it* as heard in pronunciations of such words as *ballot, custom, landed, horses*.

The (r) in final position as in *star* (stär) and before a consonant as in *heart* (härt) is regularly indicated in the respellings, but pronunciations without (r) are unquestionably reputable. Standard British is much like the speech of Eastern New England and the Lower South in this feature.

In a few words, such as *button* (but′n) and *sudden* (sud′n), no vowel appears in the unstressed syllable because the (n) constitutes the whole syllable.

The Word-Building Strategy

Quick Medical Terminology teaches you a strategy for word-building. The vocabulary of medicine is large and complex, but you can learn much of it by breaking down a complex term into its meaningful parts and putting together a word from those meaningful parts. Cover the column on the left and check your answers when you are done. Let's begin.

1.
All words have a word root. The *root* is the base or the foundation of the word, regardless of what other word, unit, or syllable may be attached to it.

For example: *do* is the root of un*do* and *do*ing.

What is the root of import, export, transport, and support?

port ____________________

2.
In this example, the words suffix, prefix, affix, and fixation have *fix*

root as their ____________________.

3.
What is the root in tonsill/itis, tonsill/ectomy, and tonsill/ar?

tonsil ____________________

4.
Two or more words may be combined to form a meaningful compound word. Using two or more of the following words, create some meaningful compound words:

Some suggestions:	over	stand
overhang	hang	wear
overcome	under	come
understand	grand	out
grandstand		
outcome,		
etc.		

____

____

____

Answer	Frame
	5.
yes	Is teaspoon a compound word? ____________
Two words are combined to make a meaningful compound term.	Explain your answer. ____________________ ____________________
	6.
	A word root and a whole word may form a compound word. But the root must be in its *combining form*. The root plus a vowel (a, e, i, o, u) make the combining form. Here are two compound terms, micr/o/scope and tel/e/cast.
micr tel	What are the word roots? ____________________
micr/o tel/e	What are the combining forms? ____________________
	7.
phon/o/graph gastr/o/enteric laryng/o/spasm	Underline the combining form in each of the following words: phon/o/graph gastr/o/enter/ic laryng/o/spasm
	8.
a word root plus a vowel (a, e, i, o, u)	The combining form in compound words is made up of a ____________________ plus a ____________________.
	9.
a combining form	In tel/e/graph and tel/e/phone the root plus a vowel are necessary to make these compound words. What is this special form called? ____________________ ______________
	10.
	Compound terms may be composed of which of the following? a) two or more whole words b) a whole word and a word root c) a word root combining form and a word
all three	Your answer? ____________________
	11.
combining form	Two roots may join together but one of them will be in a special form called the ____________________ ______________.

12.
What kind of words are these: microfilm and telecommunication?

compound terms

____

a combining form
(a root plus a vowel)
a whole word

What word parts are these terms made of? ________________
____
____

13.
Many medical terms are made of a combining form, a word root, and an ending. In the term micr/o/scop/ic,

micr/o — the combining form is ____________,

-ic — the ending is __________,

micr- — the root is ____________.

Is there another word root? ______________

scop- — What might it be? ____________

14.
There are two word roots in micr/o/scop/ic. The root *micr* is in the combining form because it is attached to a word that begins with a consonant. There is no need to add a vowel to the root *scop* because the ending *-ic* begins with a ______________.

vowel

15.
Build a term from the combining form electr/o, the word root stat, and the ending -ic.

electrostatic

______________ / _____ / __________ / ________

16.
In the word hydroelectric,

word root — electr is the ____________________,

word — hydro is the ________________,

ending — -ic is the ________________.

17.
Endings change the basic meaning of a root or foundation word. Examine the following sentences:

> Joe's job was blast-ing the rocks.
> Tejo was blast-ed by the cannon.

ending — The meaning of *blast* is changed by its ______________.

18.
A *suffix* is a word unit or syllable added to the end of a word or root that alters its meaning and creates a new word. In the words plant/er, plant/ed, and plant/ing, are these endings also suffixes? ___ Explain your answer.

____

____

yes
The endings added to the root changed its meaning.

19.
You can change the meaning of a word (or root) by adding a suffix. The suffix *-er* means *one who.* The word *port* means *to carry. Add* the suffix to the word root, *write* the word, and *explain* what it means.

__________ ______________________________

porter
one who carries

20.
When *-able* is added to the end of *read* it forms the new word *readable.* -Able is a meaningful unit added to the end of a word, creating a new word. So -able is a __________.

suffix

21.
A *prefix* is a meaningful unit joined to the beginning of a word or root that creates a new term. In the words im/plant, sup/plant, and trans/plant, the prefixes are ________, ________, and ________.

im-, sup-,
trans-

22.
In the word dis/please, *dis-* is a meaningful unit that comes before the word and changes the meaning of please; dis- is a ________.

prefix

23.
Meaningful units that go in front of a root are called prefixes. Meaningful units placed after a root are called suffixes.

Label the units in this word:

un-	manage	-able
________	________	________

prefix root suffix

24.
A suffix or a prefix is called a meaningful unit because when it is attached or added to a root or word it changes the __________ of the __________.

meaning
word

Our suggestion:
-itis is a word unit added to the end of a word altering its meaning.

25.
Explain why *-itis* in tendonitis is called a suffix.

____

____

OK, let's review what you've covered.

26.
The fundamental base from which meaningful terms grow or are formed is called the ______________.

root

27.
A meaningful word or unit placed in front of a root or word is a ______________.

prefix

28.
A syllable or word part joined to the end of a root or word that changes its meaning is a ______________.

suffix

29.
When a vowel (a, e, i, o, u) is added to a word root, the word part resulting is called the ______________ ______________.

combining form

30.
When two or more word roots combine to form a meaningful word, that word is called a ______________.

compound word

List of Illustrations

(All illustrations created by Sakrantip Blazicek of Ocala, Florida.)

1 Basic Word Roots and Common Suffixes

In Chapter 1 you will work with basic word roots and a handful of common suffixes. (These are listed in the Mini-Glossary below.) You'll examine many compound medical terms and discover meanings for all the parts. You'll practice adding various endings to roots and combining forms. By study and practice you'll make more than 30 meaningful medical terms.

Mini-Glossary

Root Words

acr/o (*extremities*)
cardi/o (*heart*)
cyan/o (*blue*)
cyt/o (*cell*)
dermat/o, derm/o (*skin*)
duoden/o (*duodenum*)
electr/o (*electrical*)
eti/o (*cause*)
gastr/o (*stomach*)
gram/o (*record*)
leuk/o (*white*)
megal/o (*enlarged*)
path/o (*disease*)

Suffixes

-algia (*pain*)
-ectomy (*excision of*)
-itis (*inflammation of*)
-ologist (*one who studies, a specialist*)
-ology (*study of*)
-osis, -a, -y (*condition of, usually abnormal*)
-ostomy (*forming a new opening*)
-otomy (*incision into*)
-tome (*instrument that cuts*)

1.
Acr/o means extremities (arms, legs, and the head). To refer to one or more extremities, physicians use words containing
__________ / ______.

acr/o

2.
Extremities are the parts of the body farthest from the center of the body. You could say these parts are located on the extreme ends of the main body. What parts are they?
____

arms, legs, and head

3.
Extremities in the human body are also known as limbs. When referring to the arms or legs we use the word acr/o. What term could designate the head as an extremity?
____

acr, acr/o

4.
When you read a term containing acr or acr/o (the combining form), it should make you think of ______________.

extremities or limbs

5.
Each of the terms acr/o/megaly, acr/o/cyan/osis, and acr/o/dermat/itis has a common word root that refers to what parts of the body? __________, __________, and __________.

arms, legs, head

Write the combining form of the word root meaning extremities.
____

acr/o

6.
Megal/o means enlarged or oversized. A word containing megal/o means the part of the body or organ is ______________ __________.

oversized, big, or enlarged

7.
The suffix -*y* denotes a condition, usually abnormal. Acr/o/megal/y means the patient's abnormal condition involves extremities that are ______________________________.

oversized or enlarged

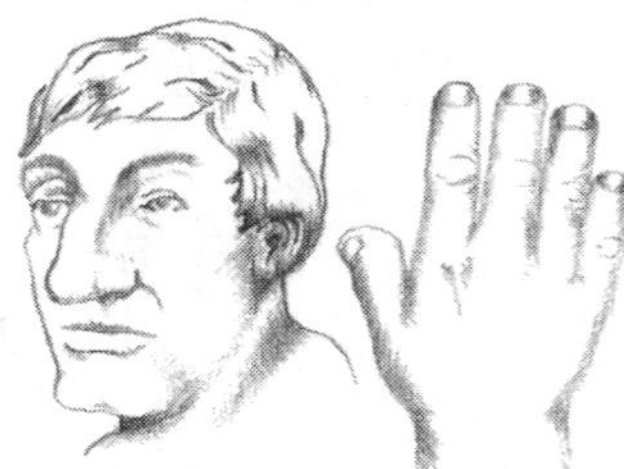

Figure 1.1 Acromegaly

acr/o/megal/y acromegaly ak rō meg′ a lē	8. Figure 1.1 on page 2 shows a man with abnormally large hands and head. The term that describes this man's abnormal condition is ________ / ____ / ______________ / ____.
acro/megaly	9. Occasionally you may see a person with very large hands, feet, nose, and/or chin. The abnormal condition may be __________ / ________________.
	10. Here are new suffixes/root words: *-ologist* means one who studies, a specialist *-itis* means inflammation of (something) *dermat/o* refers to the skin.
skin	A dermat/ologist is a specialist in the field of medicine who specializes in treating disease of the ________________.
inflammation of the skin	Dermat/itis means ________________________________.
	Underline the word root in the following medical terms. Now, circle the suffix in each term.
Dermat(itis) Dermat(ologist)	Dermatitis Dermatologist
acr/o/dermat/itis acrodermatitis ak rō der′ ma tī′ tis	11. Acrodermatitis is a term meaning inflammation of the skin of the extremities. A person displaying red, inflamed hands may have a condition of ________ / ____ / ______________ / ____________.
acrodermatitis	12. A patient may experience an inflammatory condition of her hands and lower arms. The physician may describe this abnormal condition as ________________.
inflammation of extremities skin	13. Remembering that the term acrodermatitis means inflammation of the skin of the extremities, explain the following: -itis is a suffix that means ________________. acr/o refers to ______________. dermat is the root for ______________.

14.
Cyan/o means blue or blueness. The suffix *-osis* denotes an abnormal condition. Cyan/osis means an abnormal condition of blueness.

abnormal blueness of the extremities

What do you think acr/o/cyan/osis means? ______________________

cyan or cyan/o

The part of the medical term that tells you the color blue is present is ______________.

-osis

The part of the medical term denoting that an abnormal condition exists is the suffix __________.

15.

-osis

To denote an abnormal condition, use the suffix __________.

condition
extremities

Acrocyanosis may be defined as the abnormal ______________ of blueness of the ______________.

16.

acr/o/cyan/osis
acrocyanosis
ak rō sī ə nō′sis

Blueness of the extremities is usually due to a reduced amount of oxygen supply to the hands and feet and can be considered normal in a newborn. If the lungs don't take in enough oxygen or the heart doesn't pump enough good blood around the body, the patient's hands and feet may exhibit an abnormal condition described as ________ / _____ / __________ / __________.

17.

acrocyanosis

When the lungs cannot move enough oxygen into the blood because of asthma, blueness of the extremities may result. This is another cause of ______________.

18.

the abnormal condition of blueness of the extremities

Acrocyanosis means ______________________________________.

19.

-osis

Dermat/osis denotes an abnormal skin condition. The suffix that means abnormal condition is ______________.

20.

cyan/osis
cyanosis
sī ə nō′sis

The suffix *-osis* means (usually abnormal) condition. Now, build a term that means an abnormal condition of blueness: __________ / __________.

dermat/osis dermatosis der ma tō′sis	21. Build a term meaning an abnormal skin condition: ________________ / ____________.
skin	22. The Greek word *tomos* means a piece cut off. From this word we have many words that refer to cutting: ectomy (cut out), otomy (cut into), -tome (an instrument that cuts). A dermatome is an instrument that cuts ____________.
dermat/ome dermatome derm′ə tōm	23. A dermatome is a surgical instrument. When a physician wants a thin slice of a patient's skin for a skin graft, the doctor asks for a ________________ / ____________.
an abnormal condition of bluish discoloration of the skin	24. Dermat, dermat/o refer to the skin. Cyan/o/derm/a means ____.
a disease or abnormal condition of the skin	Dermat/osis means ________________________________ ________________.
cyan/o/derm/a cyanoderma sī ə nō der′mä	25. Cyanoderma sometimes occurs when people swim too long in cold water. If a patient has a bluish discoloration of the skin, for any reason, the person may exhibit ____________ / _____ / ____________ / _____.
leuk or leuk/o	26. *Leuk/o* means white or abnormally white. In the term leuk/o/derm/a, the part that means white is ________________.
a condition of white skin, or abnormally white skin	27. Leukoderma means ____.
leuk/o/derm/a leukoderma lo͞o kō der′ mä	28. Some people have much less color in their skin than is normal. Their skin is white. They may have ____________ / _____ / ____________ / _____.

29.
Cyt/o refers to a cell or cells. *-ology* is a suffix that means the study of.

What does cyt/ology mean? ______________________________

the study of cells

30.
There are several kinds of cells in blood. One kind is the leuk/o/cyte.
A leukocyte is a ______________________________.

white blood cell

31.
There are several different kinds of cells in the bloodstream. When a physician wants to know how many infection-fighting white blood cells are circulating, the doctor asks the lab technician to count the ____________ / _____ /cytes.

leuk/o/cyt/e
leukocyte
lo͞o′ kō sīt

32.
-emia is a suffix meaning blood. When a person's blood contains far too many white blood cells, it may indicate a condition sometimes described as a cancer of the blood. A term meaning literally *white blood* is ____________ / ____________.

leuk/emia
leukemia
lo͞o kē′ mē ə

33.
In the term *acromegaly,* the combining form used for extremities is ____________, the word root for oversized is ______________, and the suffix meaning *condition of* is ______.

acr/o
megal
y

34.
Now try this. *Cardi/o* means heart. Another suffix meaning condition of is *-a*. What does megal/o/cardi/a mean? ______________
____

a condition of oversized heart, or enlargement of the heart

35.
When any muscle exercises, it gets larger. If the heart muscle overexercises, an enlarged condition of the heart may occur.
It is described as
______________ / _____ / ____________ / ________.

megal/o/card/ia
megalocardia
meg ə lō kär′ dē ä

36.

When the heart muscle doesn't receive an adequate supply of oxygen, the heart may beat more often. Inadequate oxygen makes the heart work harder and may lead to an enlarged heart described as ______________________.

megalocardia or cardiomegaly

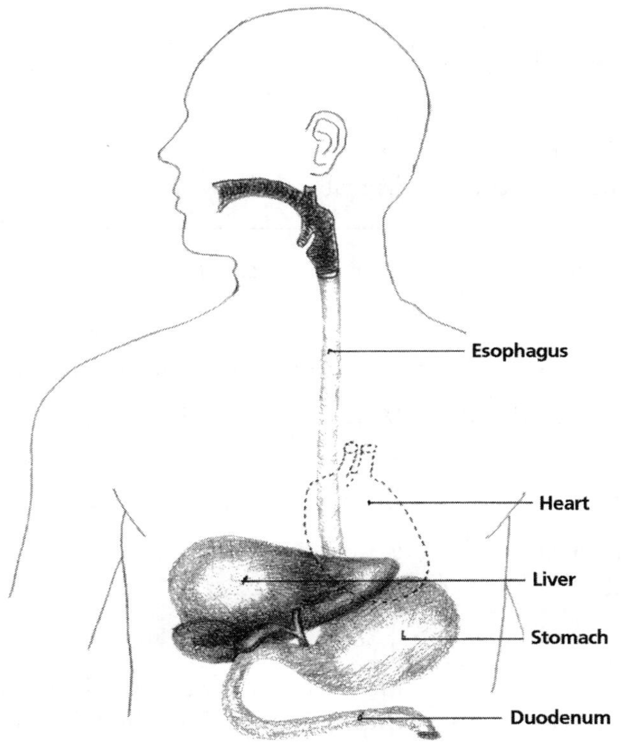

Figure 1.2 The Upper Digestive Tract (and Heart)

The digestive tract begins with the oral cavity. The teeth pulverize ingested food and soften it. The action of the tongue moves the partly digested food into the *esophagus* by swallowing. Then strong muscular contractions move the food to the *stomach*. In the stomach the food is further processed mechanically and chemically. Then it passes into the highly coiled intestine. The first part of the intestine is called the *duodenum*.

esophagus (esophag/o) stomach (gastr/o)
duodenum (duoden/o) heart (cardi/o)

Answers	Frames
megal/o/gastr/ia megalogastria meg ə lō gas′ trē ä or gastr/o/megal/y gastromegaly gas′ trō meg′ a lē	37. Try this one. *Gastr* is the word root for stomach. When the stomach enlarges so that it crowds other organs, an undesirable condition exists known as __________ (enlarged) / _____ / __________ (stomach) /ia. or __________ (stomach) / _____ / __________ (enlarged) /y.
oversized heart, or enlargement of the heart	38. Megalocardia means ______________________________.
(the same thing)	What does cardiomegaly mean? ____________________
	39. The suffix *-itis* means inflammation.
inflammation of the heart	What does carditis mean? ____________________
stomach	Both gastr-, gastr/o mean ____________________.
inflammation of the stomach	Gastritis means ______________________________.
	40. Here's a quick review. Using the suggested answers, write the meaning of each of the following terms. SUGGESTED ANSWERS: abnormal condition of; blueness; cell; cutting instrument; enlarged, oversized; extremities; heart; inflammation of; skin; stomach; white
extremities	acr/o ____________________
blueness	cyan/o ____________________
white	leuk/o ____________________
stomach	gastr/o ____________________
cell	cyt/o ____________________
heart	cardi/o ____________________

enlarged, oversized	megal/o ________
skin	derm/o, dermat/o ________
abnormal condition of	-osis (-a, -y) ________
inflammation of	-itis ________
cutting instrument	-tome ________

41.
Now build a medical term for each of the following:

acro/megal/y	a condition of oversized extremities ________ / ________ / ____ extremities oversized
leuko/cyte	a white cell ________ / ________
dermat/itis	inflammation of the skin ________ / ________
megalo/cardi/a or cardio/megal/y	a condition of enlarged heart ________ / ________ / ____

42.
Let's have a change of pace here. Professional health workers use some special words to talk about illness and sick people. Here are just a few you'll find very useful. Read each definition. Then underline a key word or words to help you remember the meaning of the term.

It's up to you, of course, but here are some key words.

<u>sickness</u>, <u>illness</u>	*Disease* is a condition in which bodily health is impaired. It means sickness or illness.
<u>exhibition</u>, <u>display</u>, <u>evidence</u>	*Manifestation* is proof of impaired bodily health. It's a display, exhibition, or physical evidence of disease.
<u>changes</u> (structural and functional)	*Pathology* is the scientific study of changes in the human body (structural and functional) produced by disease.
<u>causes</u> (ētēology)	*Etiology* is the scientific study of causes of disease.

You may refer to the definitions if you need help answering the next few frames.

43.
If a physician says that a patient's disease is of unknown etiology, what would that mean to you? ________
____
____

The cause of the patient's disease is not yet known (and may remain unknown).

44.
Another word for disease is ________________.

sickness, illness

45.
Manifestation is a display, or ________________, of disease.

evidence, or exhibition

46.
Etiology is the scientific study of ________________ of disease.

causes

47.
Pathology is the scientific study of ________________ and ________________ changes in the body produced by ________________.

structural
functional
disease

48.
Select the best term for each definition. Write your choice in the space provided.

pathology etiology manifestation disease

Another term for illness or sickness is ________________. — disease

Evidence, or proof, of disease is ________________. — manifestation

The study of causes of disease is ________________. — etiology

The scientific study of changes in the body produced by disease is ________________. — pathology

49.
The suffix *-ology* means the study of, the suffix *-ologist* means one who studies (and becomes an expert). One who studies structural and functional changes in the body produced by disease is a ________________ / ________________.

path/ologist
pathologist
path ol′ ə jist

50.
Some physicians specialize in heart disease. The specialist who determines that a heart is deformed is a
________________ / ________________.
heart specialist

cardi/ologist
cardiologist
kär dē ol′ ə jist

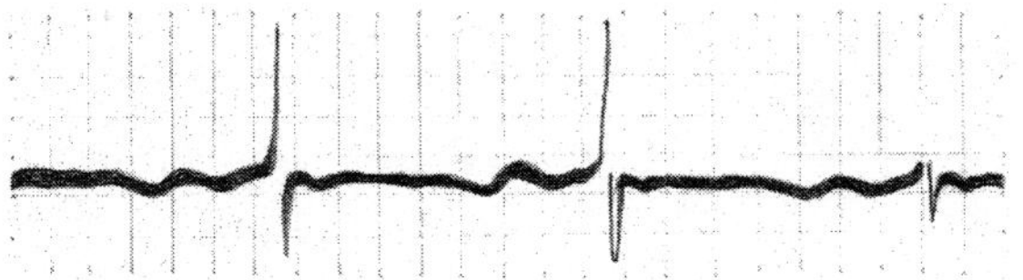

Figure 1.3 Electrocardiogram (ECG)

Electrocardiography is a method of recording electrical currents traversing the heart muscle just prior to each heartbeat. An electrocardiogram (ECG) is a graphic record of heart action currents that are obtained by electrocardiography.

51.
A heart doctor who reads an electr/o/cardi/o/gram (a record of electrical impulses generated by the heart) is a specialist in heart problems or a ________________ / ________________.

cardiologist

52.
Complete the meaning of electr/o/cardi/o/gram:

Gram means a record or recording, electr/o means ______________ ______________________________________ ______________________________________,

and cardi/o means ________________.

a record of electrical waves given off by the heart (or equivalent)

heart

53.
The electr/o/cardi/o/gram is a record obtained by electr/o/cardi/o/graph/y. A technician can learn electrocardiography, but it takes a cardiologist to read the

______________ / ______ / __________ / _____ / __________.
(electrical) (heart) (record)

electr/o/cardi/o/gram
electrocardiogram
ē lek′ trō kär′ dē ə gram

54.
A physician specialist can look at a report that looks like this

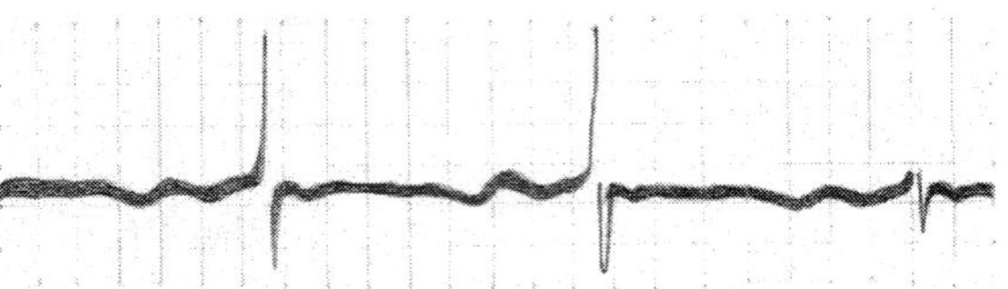

Figure 1.4 Electrocardiogram (ECG)

cardiologist
electrocardiogram

and learn something about a patient's heart function. This specialist is probably a ________________ and can read an ________________.
(ECG)

cardi/algia
cardialgia
kär dē al′ jē a (There is no need to add a vowel to the root cardi because -algia begins with a vowel.)

55.
The suffix *-algia* means pain. Form a word that means heart pain:
________________ / ________________.
heart pain

cardialgia

56.
When a patient complains of pain in the heart, the symptom is known medically as ________________.

stomach
-algia

57.
Gastralgia means pain in the stomach.

Gastr is the root for ________________.

The suffix for pain is ________________.

stomach
to cut out, excise, or remove surgically

58.
Gastr/ectomy means excision (removal) of all or part of the stomach. *Gastr* means ________________.

The suffix *-ectomy* means ________________
________________.

gastr/ectomy gastrectomy gas trek′ tō mē	59. When a patient's stomach ulcer perforates, the surgeon may need to remove part of the stomach. The medical term for the procedure is ______________ / ________________. (stomach) (excision of)
gastrectomy	60. Cancer of the stomach may require a surgeon to remove all or part of the patient's stomach. This procedure is a ________________.
gastr/itis gastritis gas trī′ tis	61. Form a word that means inflammation of the stomach: ______________ / ____________.
duoden/um duodenum do͞o ōd′ nəm (or do͞o ō dē′ nəm)	62. The stomach empties its contents into the first section of the intestine, called the duodenum. *Duoden* is the word root for ________________.
gastr	What is the root for stomach? ____________
stomach and duodenum	63. The suffix *-ostomy* means a procedure to form a new opening. Gastr/o/duoden/ostomy means forming a new opening between the ________________ and ________________.
gastr/o/duoden/ ostomy gastroduodenostomy gas′ trō do͞o ō de nos′ tō mē	64. A surgeon may need to remove a portion of a diseased stomach. If the natural connection is removed, then the surgeon must form a new opening between the stomach and duodenum. This procedure is called __________ / _____ / ______________ / ______________.
a surgical procedure to form a new opening between the stomach and duodenum	65. When an abnormal condition exists between the stomach and the duodenum, a surgeon may need to perform a gastroduodenostomy, which means ____ ____ ____.

66.
The suffix -ectomy means excision of; -ostomy means forming a new opening. The form *-otomy* means incision into. A duoden/otomy is an incision into the ________.

duodenum
dū ō dē′ num

67.
The suffix for incision into is ________.

-otomy

If a physician makes an incision into the wall of the duodenum, the doctor has performed a ________ / ________.

duoden/otomy
duodenotomy
do͞o od ə not′ ə mē

68.
The suffix for inflammation is ________.

-itis

The word for inflammation of the duodenum is ________ / ________.

duoden/itis
duodenitis
do͞o od ə nī′ tis

69.
Duoden/al means of or pertaining to the duodenum.

-al is a suffix meaning of, or pertaining to. Therefore matern/al means ________ and patern/al means ________.

of, or pertaining to, mother; of, or pertaining to, father

70.
In the sentence "Duodenal carcinoma was present," the word meaning of, or pertaining to, the duodenum is ________ / ________.

duoden/al
duodenal
do͞o ō dē′ nəl

71.
The suffix -ostomy means making a new opening. The word to form a new opening into the duodenum is ________ / ________.

duoden/ostomy
duodenostomy
do͞o od ə nos′ tō mē

72.
Here's one for you to figure out. A duodenostomy can be formed in more than one manner. If it is formed with the stomach, it is called a ________.
stomach duodenum new opening

gastroduodenostomy

73.
The suffix for forming a new opening is ________.

-ostomy

74.

Let's review what you've covered. Using the suggested answers, write the meaning of each of the following terms.

SUGGESTED ANSWERS:

blueness	duodenum
cell	electrical
cause(s)	enlarged, oversized
changes due to disease	record of

Answer	Term
duodenum	duoden/o ______
changes due to disease	path/o ______
record of	gram/o ______
cell	cyt/o ______
electric	electr/o ______
cause	eti/o ______
enlarged, oversized	megal/o ______
blueness	cyan/o ______

75.

Now try it with the suffixes you just learned.

SUGGESTED ANSWERS:

(abnormal) condition of	incision into
cutting instrument	inflammation of
form a new opening	of, or pertaining to
one who studies, specializes in	pain

Answer	Term
of, or pertaining to	-al ______
inflammation of	-itis ______
(abnormal) condition	-osis, -a, -y ______
form a new opening	-ostomy ______
cutting instrument	-tome ______
incision into	-otomy ______
pain	-algia ______
one who studies	-ologist ______

76.

Now build some new words.

cyan/osis

A condition of blueness is ____________ / ____________.
(blueness) (condition)

path/ologist

One who studies bodily changes produced by disease is a ____________ / ____________.
(changes in the body) (one who studies)

duoden/ostomy

A surgical procedure that forms a new opening in the duodenum is a ____________ / ____________.
(duodenum) (form a new opening)

eti/o/logic/al

A term meaning of, or pertaining to, the study of causes of disease is ____________ / ______ / ____________ / ____________.
(causes of disease) (the study of) (pertaining to)

77.

While working through Chapter 1, you formed the following new medical terms. Read them one at a time and pronounce each aloud several times until you can articulate each term clearly and correctly. If a friend pronounces each term for you, could you spell it correctly? Try it.

acrocyanosis (ak rō sī ə nō′ sis)
acrodermatitis (ak rō der′ ma tī′tis)
acromegaly (ak rō meg′ a lē)
cardialgia (kär dē al′ jē a)
cardiologist (kär dē ol′ ə jist)
carditis (kär dī′ tis)
cyanoderma (sī ə nō der′ mä)
cyanosis (sī ə nō′ sis)
cytology (sī tol′ ə jē)
dermatologist (der ma tol′ ə jist)
dermatome (derm′ ə tōm)
dermatosis (der ma tō′ sis)
disease (diz ēz′)
duodenal (do͞o ō dē′ nəl)
electrocardiogram (ē lek′ trō kär′ dē ə gram)
etiological (ē′ tē ō loj′ i kəl)
gastralgia (gas tral′ jē a)
gastrectomy (gas trek′ tō mē)
gastritis (gas trī′ tis)
gastroduodenostomy (gas′ trō do͞o ō de nos′ tō mē)
leukemia (lo͞o kē′ mē ə)
leukocyte (lo͞o′ kō sīt)
leukoderma (lo͞o kō der′ mä)
manifestation (man′ ə fes t1′ shən)
megalocardia (meg ə lō kär′ dē ä)
megalogastria (meg ə lō gas′ trē ä)
pathologist (path ol′ ə jist)
pathology (path ol′ ə jē)

Before going on to Chapter 2, take the Chapter 1 Self-Test that follows.

Chapter 1 Self-Test

Part 1

From the list of definitions on the right, select the correct meaning for each of the terms in the left-hand column. Write the letter in the space provided.

_____ 1. Megalocardia
_____ 2. Cardiology
_____ 3. Duodenostomy
_____ 4. Leukemia
_____ 5. Dermatologist
_____ 6. Electrocardiography
_____ 7. Acromegaly
_____ 8. Gastritis
_____ 9. Dermatome
_____ 10. Manifestation
_____ 11. Gastroduodenostomy
_____ 12. Etiology
_____ 13. Acrocyanosis
_____ 14. Pathologist
_____ 15. Gastralgia

a. Study of, or pertaining to, causes (of disease)
b. A specialist in the field of skin diseases
c. A condition of blueness of the extremities
d. Enlargement of the heart
e. A surgical procedure forming a new opening in the duodenum
f. Display, evidence of disease
g. One who specializes in the study of structural and functional changes in the body
h. Pain in the stomach
i. Inflammation of the stomach
j. Recordings of electrical waves of the heart
k. An abnormal condition of enlarged extremities
l. A surgical instrument for cutting skin
m. A surgical operation to make a new opening between the stomach and duodenum
n. The study of disease of the heart
o. An abnormal condition of too many white blood cells

Part 2

Write a medical term for each of the following:

1. Impaired bodily health __________
2. Bluish discoloration of the skin __________
3. White cell __________
4. Oversized or enlarged stomach __________
5. Evidence of disease __________
6. The study of causes of an illness __________
7. Excision or removal of the stomach __________
8. Pertaining to the duodenum __________
9. Generalized condition of blueness __________
10. Heart pain __________
11. Inflammation of the heart __________
12. An abnormal condition of white skin __________
13. Inflammation of the skin of the extremities __________
14. Study of cell(s) __________
15. An abnormal condition of the skin __________

ANSWERS

Part 1	***Part 2***
1. d	1. disease
2. n	2. cyanoderma
3. e	3. leukocyte
4. o	4. megalogastria
5. b	5. manifestation
6. j	6. etiology
7. k	7. gastrectomy
8. i	8. duodenal
9. l	9. cyanosis
10. f	10. cardialgia

11. m
12. a
13. c
14. g
15. h

11. carditis
12. leukoderma
13. acrodermatitis
14. cytology
15. dermatosis

2 More Word Roots, Suffixes, and Prefixes

In Chapter 2 you will cover more sophisticated terms, word roots, and suffixes, and you'll begin using prefixes. Teaching sequences in this unit aim to expand your learning by combining words you covered in Chapter 1 with some new ones. We introduced new ideas as well as useful medical terms to improve retention and make your practice exercises interesting. Now, let's get started.

Mini-Glossary

Root Words

aden/o (*gland*)
arthr/o (*joint*)
carcin/o (*malignancy*)
cele/o, o/cele (*hernia*)
cephal/o (*head*)
chondr/o (*cartilage*)
cost/o (*ribs*)
dent/o (*tooth*)
emes/is (*vomiting*)
hist/o (*tissue*)
laryng/o (*larynx*)
lip/o (*fat*)
malac/o (*soft*)
morph/o (*structure* of)
muc/o (*mucus*)
onc/o (*tumor*)
ost/o, oste/o (*bone*)
plast/o (*repair*)
trach/e (*trachea*)
troph/o (*development*)

Prefixes

en-, endo- (*in, inside, within*)
ex-, ex/o- (*outside, out*)
hyper- (*excessive*)
hypo- (*under*)
inter- (*between*)

Suffixes

-al, -ar, -ic (*of, or pertaining to*)
-oid (*resembling*)
-oma (*tumor*)
-ism (*medical condition, disease*)

Before you begin Chapter 2, complete the Review Sheet for Chapter 1. It will help you get a running start as you continue your studying. You'll find review sheets beginning on page 261.

1.
Examine the terms hyper/trophy, hyper/emia, and hyper/emesis. *Hyper-* means excessive, more than normal amount. Hyper- placed in front of trophy, emia, and emesis changes the meaning of the terms. Therefore, hyper- is a ________________ (prefix/suffix?).

prefix

2.
Hyper/thyroid/ism is a medical condition of the thyroid gland resulting in excessive thyroid gland activity. The prefix expressing higher than normal activity of the thyroid gland is ______________.

hyper

3.
The suffix *-ism* indicates there is a medical condition involving some specified thing or body part. In the case of hyper/thyroid/ism the medical condition involves what body part? ________________

thyroid gland

4.
Hyper- means something is excessive. Thyroid tells you what part is involved. The suffix -ism means there is a resulting medical condition.

In your words, explain the meaning of the term hyper/thyroid/ism.
____
____
____

Here's a suggestion: Hyperthyroidism means the patient has a medical condition resulting from excessive activity of the thyroid gland.

5.
Emesis is a word that means vomiting. A word that means excessive vomiting is ______________ / ________________.

Gallbladder attacks can cause excessive vomiting. This, too, is called ________________.

hyper/emesis
hyperemesis
hī per em′ ə sis

hyperemesis

6.
Hyper/trophy means overdevelopment; *troph/o* comes from the Greek word for nourishment. Note the connection between nourishment and development. Overdevelopment is called
______________ / ______________ /y.
a condition of excessive development

hyper/troph/y
hypertrophy
hī per′ trō fē

Muscles also can overdevelop or ________________.
(a verb form)

hypertrophy

Answer	Frame
hypertrophy	7. Many organs can overdevelop. If the heart overdevelops, the condition is called cardiac ________________.
hypo-	8. The prefix *hypo-* is just the opposite of hyper–. The prefix for under or less than normal is ________________.
skin skin	9. Derm/o refers to the ________________. The suffix -ic means of, or pertaining to. Hypo/derm/ic means pertaining to under the ________________.
hypo/derm/ic hypodermic hī pō der′ mik	10. A hypodermic needle is short because it goes just under the skin. A shot given superficially is administered with a ____________ / ____________ / __________ needle. (under) (skin) (pertaining to)
aden/itis adenitis ad ə nī′ tis	11. *Aden/o* is used in words that refer to glands. Build a word that means inflammation of a gland: ____________ / ____________. (gland) (inflammation of)
aden/ectomy adenectomy ad ə nek′ tō mē	12. Since -ectomy means excision (or surgical removal of), the word for surgical removal of a gland is ____________ / ________________. (gland) (surgical removal)
adenectomy	13. If a gland is inflammed or abnormal, part or all of it may be excised. Excision of a gland is ________________.
aden/oma adenoma ad ə nō′ mä	14. The suffix *-oma* means tumor. Form a word that means tumor of a gland: ____________ / __________.
surgical removal, or excision, of the thyroid gland	15. Try this. Sometimes the thyroid gland develops a tumor. A patient's history might read, ". . . because of the presence of a thyroid adenoma, thyroidectomy is indicated." What is a thyroid/ectomy? ____ ____

	16. The suffixes *-ic, -al,* and *-ar* mean of, or pertaining to, the attached word.
spleen	A splenic tumor is a tumor of the ________________.
tonsil	A tonsillar tumor is a tumor pertaining to the ________________.
in the duodenum	Where would you expect to find a duodenal tumor? ____________ ____________________
cancerous tumor	17. *Carcin/o* is the root for cancer. The suffix -oma means tumor. A carcinoma is a ____________________.
splenic	18. A carcinoma may occur in almost any part of the body. A cancerous tumor of the spleen is called ________________ carcinoma.
carcinoma	Cancer of the tonsil is tonsillar ________________.
of, or pertaining to	The suffixes -ic, -ar, and -al mean ____________________.
tumor	19. An adenoma is a glandular tumor; -oma means ________________.
	A lip/oma is a tumor of fatty tissue.
fat, fatty tissue	*Lip/o* is the combining form for ________________.
lip/oma lipoma li po′ ma	20. A fatty tumor is called a __________ / __________.
lip/oid lipoid lip′ oid	21. Lipoma is a fatty tumor; *-oid* is a suffix meaning like or resembling. Using the word root for fatty tissue, build a term that means fatlike, or resembling fat: __________ / __________.
lip/oid	22. The word lipoid is used in chemistry and pathology. It describes a substance that looks like fat, dissolves like fat, but is not fat. Cholesterol is an alcohol that resembles fat; therefore, cholesterol is a __________ / __________ substance. (fat) (like)

23.

muc/oid mucoid my$\overline{oo}$′ koid	*Muc/oid* means resembling mucus. There is a substance in connective tissue that resembles mucus. This is called a ___________ / ___________ substance.

24.

resembling mucus	There is a protein in the body that is said to be mucoid in nature. Mucoid means ______________________________.

25.

mucoid	A substance that resembles mucus is best described as _______________.
lipoid	A substance resembling fatty tissue is called a _______________ substance.

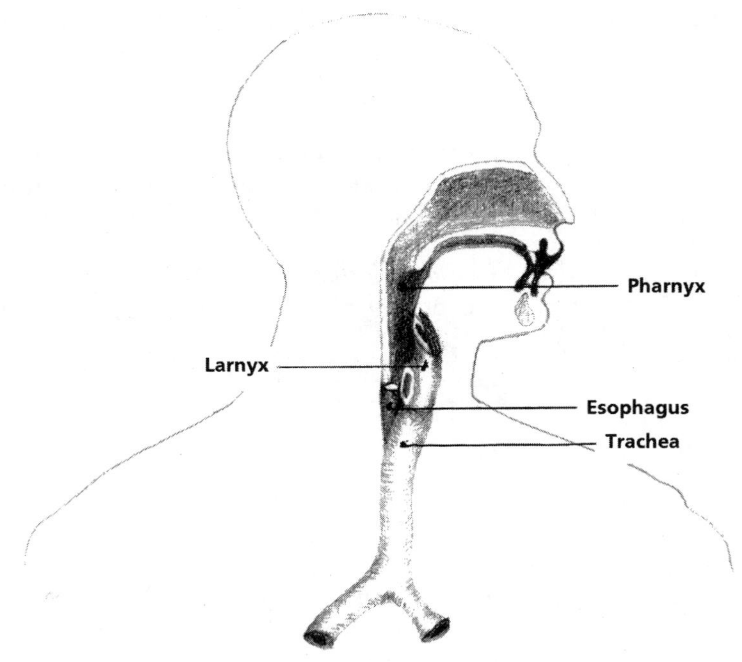

Figure 2.1 The Upper Respiratory Tract

The respiratory tract conducts oxygen-rich air to the lungs where oxygen can be readily absorbed by the blood. It removes carbon dioxide–laden air to the external atmosphere. The *pharynx* filters and warms the air we breathe and conducts it into the *larynx*. The larynx protects against inadvertent inhaling of solid matter and contains the vocal cords, the mechanism of sound production. Leading from the larynx is the windpipe, more correctly known as the *trachea*.

pharynx (pharyng/o) trachea (trache/o)
larynx (laryng/o)

26.
The larynx or *voice box* contains the vocal cords. *Laryng/o* is the combining form for building words referring to the voice box, also called the ______________.

larynx

Build a term meaning inflammation of the larynx:
______________ / ____________.

laryng/itis
laryngitis
lair an jī′ tis

27.
After a bad cold, a patient may develop laryngitis, which means ______________________________.

inflammation of the larynx

28.
Now, you'll add a few new suffixes to your growing vocabulary. An obstruction of the colon may require a new opening into the colon that will be *permanent*.

Col, col/o refer to the colon, or large bowel. The suffix *-ostomy* means a permanent artificial opening into.

Col/ostomy means ______________________________
______________________________.

(kō los′ tō mē)
permanent artificial opening into the colon

29.
The suffix for a permanent opening is ______________.

-ostomy

30.
Take a look at Figure 2.1. An obstruction of the trachea makes breathing very difficult, or even impossible. In an emergency, a physician may make an incision into the windpipe to permit a free flow of air to the patient's lungs.

Trache, trache/o refer to the trachea, or *windpipe*. The suffix -otomy means incision into, or a *temporary* opening.

Trache/otomy means ______________________________
______________________________.

(trā kē ot′ ō mē)
an incision into, or temporary opening into, the trachea, or windpipe

31.
The suffix meaning a temporary opening, or incision into, is ________.

-otomy

32.
Which suffix would you use to indicate creation of a permanent artificial opening? ________

-ostomy

Which suffix means making an incision into, or creating a temporary opening? ________

-otomy

32.
Colostomy means ________
________.

creation of a permanent opening into the colon

Tracheotomy means ________
________.

incision into, or temporary opening into, the trachea

34.
Time for a quick review. Using the suggested answers, write a meaning for each of the following word roots.

SUGGESTED ANSWERS:

fat, fatty	mucus
larynx	skin
cancer, malignant	spleen

lip/o ________ — fat, fatty
splen/o ________ — spleen
derm/o ________ — skin
laryng/o ________ — larynx
muc/o ________ — mucus
carcin/o ________ — cancer, malignant

35.
Now do the same with the following suffixes.

SUGGESTED ANSWERS:

incision into, temporary opening	a new (permanent) opening into
like, or resembling	development
of or pertaining to	vomiting
tumor	excision of

-trophy ________ — development
-ectomy ________ — excision of

incision into, temporary opening	-otomy ______
a permanent surgical opening into	-ostomy ______
of, or pertaining to	-ic, -ar, -al ______
like, or resembling	-oid ______
vomiting	-emesis ______
tumor	-oma ______

36.
Complete the following:

under, less	Hypo- is a prefix meaning ______.
over, excessive	Hyper- is a prefix meaning ______.

37.
Build a medical term for each of the following:

muc/oid	resembling mucus ______ (mucus) / ______ (like)
splen/ic	pertaining to the spleen ______ (spleen) / ______ (of the)
aden/ectomy	excision of a gland ______ (gland) / ______ (excision of)
hyper/trophy	overdevelopment ______ (excessive) / ______ (development)
hypo/derm/ic	under the skin ______ (under) / ______ (skin) / ______ (pertaining to)
laryng/ostomy	permanent opening into the larynx ______ (larynx) / ______ (permanent)

38.
Here are two terms to define.

a condition of excess development, oversized	Hypertrophy means ______ ______.
of, or pertaining to, under the skin	Hypodermal means ______ ______.

This is a good place to stop and take a short break.

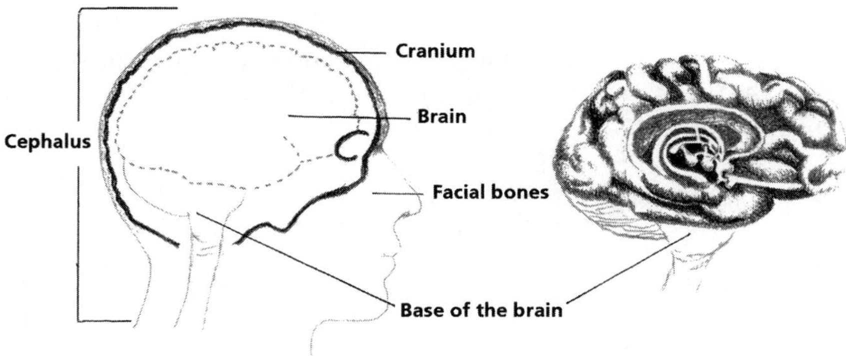

Figure 2.2 The Head

Cephalus is a term that refers to the entire head. It is composed of both the cranium and facial bones. The *cranium* (or skull) is a bony vault protecting the contents of the head. The face is the front portion of the head and includes the eyes, nose, mouth, forehead, cheeks, and chin. The cranium encloses the *cerebrum,* also known as the brain. The brain is the center of sensory awareness and movement, emotions, rational thought and behavior, foresight and planning, memory, speech, language, and interpretation of language.

cephalus, head including skull and facial bones (cephal/o)
cranium (crani/o)
cerebrum (cerebr/o)

Use the illustration of the head to help you with the frames that follow.

39.
Welcome back. At this stage of word-building, students sometimes find they have one big headache. Both ceph/algia and cephal/algia mean pain in the head. The combining form and root for head are ________________ and ________________.

cephal/o
ceph

40.
To indicate pain we use -algia. Any headache may be called
________________ / ________________ or
head pain
________________ / ________________.
head ache

ceph/algia or cephal/algia

cephalalgia (sef ə lal′ jē ä)

Answer	Frame
cephalalgia and cephalgia	41. The word root and combining form for head is *ceph, cephal/o.* Two words for pain in the head are ______________ ______________.
headache	42. Cephalalgia means ______________.
of, or pertaining to, the head	Cephal/ic means ______________ ______________.
cephal/ic cephalic sə fal′ ik	43. A case history reporting head wounds due to an accident might read, "______________ / ________ lacerations were present."
cephalic	44. A tumor located on the head might be noted as a ______________ tumor.

Prefix	Meaning
en-, endo-	in, inside, within
ex-, exo-	out, outside completely

Use the table to help with the items that follow.

Answer	Frame
inside the head (the brain)	45. Cephal/o means head. What does *en*cephal/o mean? ______________.
brain	46. Since the brain is enclosed inside the head's bony vault, encephal/o means the organ inside the head, or the ______________.
	47. Using the word root for head, build words meaning the following:
encephal/itis en sef ə lī′ tis	inflammation of the brain ______________ (brain) / ______________ (inflammation of)
encephal/oma en sef′ ə lō′ mä	brain tumor ______________ (brain) / ______________ (tumor of).
inflammation within the heart	48. What does endocarditis mean? ______________ ______________

49.
Refer to the table in question 44 for help. Select a prefix meaning out, or completely outside of: ______________________.
en-, endo- or ex-, exo-

ex-, exo-

50.
Exo/genous means originating completely outside of an organ or part. *Genous* takes its meaning from a Latin word meaning to produce or originate.

What part of the term means completely outside of? __________

exo-

Something originating completely outside of an organism, cell, or organ is called ________ / ______________.
outside / produced or originating

exo/genous
ex′ oj′ ə nus

Now build a word that indicates something is produced or originates from within a cell or organism:
__________ / ______________.
within / produced or originating

endo/genous
en′ doj′ ə nus

51.
Try these. Here are some common English words often used in the medical world. Write what each means.

hale (breathe) cise (cut) spire (breathe)

Exhale means ______________________.

breathe out

Excise means ______________________.

cut out

Expire means ______________________.

breathe out (It also means to die or breathe out for the last time.)

52.
Write two forms of a prefix for each of the following.

in, inside of, within __________, __________

en-, endo-

out, completely outside of __________, __________

ex-, exo-

53.
The Greek word for hernia is *kele*. From this we derive the combining forms *cele/o* or *o/cele*. Encephal/o/cele is a word meaning herniation of __________ tissue.

brain

54\.

encephal/o/cele
encephalocele
en səf′ a lō sēl

Any hernia is a protrusion of a body part or an organ from its natural cavity. Herniation is expressed by cele. A protrusion of brain tissue from its natural cavity is an ________________ / ______ / ____________.
brain (inside the head) … hernia

55\.

encephalocele

Increased fluid inside the head sometimes causes herniation at the base of the brain. Herniation of the brain in medical language is called an ________________.

56\.

a condition of softened brain tissue

Malac/ia is a word meaning soft, or softened, tissue. Encephal/o/malac/ia means ________________________________ ____.

57\.

encephal/o/malac/ia
encephalomalacia
en sef′ a lō mä la′ zhə

Malac/o is the combining form for soft, or softened. The term meaning softened brain tissue is ________________ / ____ / ____________ / ___ia___.
brain tissue … softened … a condition of

58\.

encephalomalacia

An accident causing brain injury could result in softened brain tissue, called ________________________________.

59\.

oste/itis
osteitis
os tē ī′ tis

Oste is the root referring to bone. A word meaning inflammation of the bone is ____________ / ____________.

60\.

a condition of softened bone tissue

What do you think oste/o/malac/ia means? ________________ ____

61\.

oste/o/malac/ia
osteomalacia
os′ tē ō mä lā′ zhə

Insufficient calcium in a young person's diet may lead to gradual softening and bending of bones. This disorder is called ____________ / ______ / ______________ / ________.
bone … softened … condition

62.
A disorder of the parathyroid gland can cause calcium to be withdrawn from bones. The resulting condition may be called ______________.

osteomalacia

63.
A hard outgrowth on any bone could be a bone tumor. In medical terms, it would be referred to as an ________ / ________.

oste/oma
osteoma
os tē ō′ mä

What does end/oste/oma mean? ______________________________

a tumor inside (the center canal of the bone)

64.
Arthr/o refers to joints; *plast/y* means surgical repair of. What does arthr/o/plast/y mean? ______________________________

surgical repair of a joint(s)

65.
Think of a plastic surgeon building a new nose or doing a face-lift. These are surgical repairs or restoration. When a joint has lost its ability to move, movement can sometimes be restored by an ________ / ____ / ________ / ___y___.
joint / / repair or restore / (process/procedure)

arthr/o/plast/y
arthroplasty
arth′ rō plas′ tē

66.
If a child is born without a joint, sometimes one can be formed by a surgical procedure called ________ / ________.

arthro/plasty

67.
Form a word that means inflammation of a joint: ________ / ________.
joint / inflammation of

arthr/itis
arthritis
ärth rī′ tis

68.
Now form a word that means incision into a joint: ________ / ________.
joint / temporary opening

arthr/otomy
arthrotomy
ärth rot′ ō mē

69.
The word oste/o/chondr/itis means inflammation of the bone and cartilage. The word root for cartilage must be ________________.

chondr

Oste, oste/o mean ________________.

bone

70.
Analyze oste/o/chondr/itis:

combining form for bone ________________

oste/o

word root for cartilage ________________

chondr

suffix for inflammation ________________

-itis

71.
Now put all the parts together:
________ / ____ / ________ / ________.
bone — cartilage — inflammation of

oste/o/chondr/itis
osteochondritis
os′ tē ō kon drī′ tis

What does osteochondritis mean? ________________

inflammation of bone and cartilage

72.
Chondr/ectomy means ________________.

excision of cartilage

73.
Cost/al means pertaining to the ribs. *Inter/*cost/al means pertaining to between the ribs. The prefix for between is ________________. The suffix -al means ________________.

inter-
of or pertaining to

74.
There are short strong muscles between the ribs. These muscles move the ribs during breathing and are called
________ / ________ / ________ muscles.
between — ribs

inter/cost/al
intercostal
in ter kos′ t'l

75.
One set of between-the-ribs muscles expands the rib cage when breathing in to make room for inflated lungs. When exhaling, the rib cage is made smaller by another set of ________________ muscles.
(between-the-ribs)

intercostal

76.

Answer	Frame
teeth teeth	A *dent*/ist takes care of __________. A dent/ifrice is used for cleaning __________.
spaces between the teeth	Interdental spaces means ____________________.

77.

Answer	Frame
dent/algia dentalgia den tal′ jē a	Try making a few new words. Pain in the teeth, or a toothache, is called __________ / __________.
dent/oid dentoid den′ toid	A word that means tooth-shaped or resembling a tooth is __________ / ______.

78.

Try these. Pathogenic means something that produces disease.

What is a pathogenic organism? ____________________

What does pathology mean? ____________________

Answer	Frame
(If you're not sure, look it up.)	Therefore, pathological means ____________________.

79.

Explain each of the following statements in simple language.

Answer	Frame
Excessive vomiting is evidence of a disease process.	Hyperemesis is a manifestation of a pathological condition. ____________________
A graphic representation of brain activity (EEG) is necessary to determine the cause of brain disease (or something similar in your words).	Electroencephalography (EEG) is often the first step toward a diagnosis of encephalopathy. ____________________

80.
It's time to review again. Using the suggested answers, write the meaning of each of the following terms.

SUGGESTED ANSWERS:

bone	joint
cartilage	rib
head	soft, soften
hernia	tooth, teeth

Answer	Term
joint	arthr/o ____
hernia	cele/o ____
head	cephal/o ____
cartilage	chondr/o ____
rib	cost/o ____
tooth, teeth	dent/o ____
soft, soften	malac/o ____
bone	ost-, oste-, oste/o ____

81.
These word parts are used as suffixes.

repair of (restoration or plastic surgery)

-plasty means ____.

hernia (protrusion of a body part or an organ from its natural cavity)

-cele means ____ ____.

82.
Here are some easy ones.

in, within, inside

end-, endo- is a prefix meaning ____.

out, completely outside of

ex-, exo- is a prefix meaning ____.

83.
Build a medical term for each of the following:

arthro/plasty

restoration of a joint ____ (joint) / ____ (plastic surgery of)

inter/costal

between the ribs ____ (between) / ____ (ribs)

chondro/malacia

softening of cartilage ____ (cartilage) / ____ (softened)

oste/oma

bony tumor ____ (bone) / ____ (tumor of)

encephalo/cele — herniation of the brain ______ / ______
inside the head / hernia of

dent/oid — resembling teeth ______ / ______
teeth / resembling

ceph/algia — headache ______ / ______
head / pain

arthr/otomy — incision into a joint ______ / ______
joint / temporary opening

84.

You just learned the suffix -oma, meaning tumor. Now, here are some more very useful terms often used in discussion of tumors.

Read each definition. Then underline a key word or two to help you remember what the term means.

Oncology is the branch of medicine dealing with tumors.

Morphology is the biological science dealing with the structure of an organ or part of the body.

Histology is the study of the microscopic tissues that make up a part or a structure.

Pathology is the study of changes in structure and function caused by disease.

Here are our suggestions:
tumors, branch of medicine
structure of an organ, part
microscopic tissues (of) a part
changes, caused by disease

85.

Complete each of the following statements. Look back at the definition if necessary.

tumors — Onc/o refers to ______.

tissues (of a part, organ) — Hist/o refers to ______.

changes (due to disease) — Path/o refers to ______.

structure (of an organ, part) — Morph/o refers to ______.

86.

Complete each definition.

structure — Morphology is the study of the ______ of an organ or part.

tissues — Histology is the study of microscopic ______ making up a part or structure.

tumors — Oncology is the study of ______.

changes — Pathology is the study of ______ caused by disease.

87.
Complete each of the following definitions:

One who studies the tissue *structure* under a microscope is a ________________. — histologist

A specialist in the care and treatment of patients with *tumors* is an ________________. — oncologist

One who studies the *structure* of living organisms is a ____________________. — morphologist

A specialist who studies *changes* in structure and function resulting from disease is a ________________. — pathologist

88.
Here are more than 30 medical terms you worked with in Chapter 2. Read each one. Say it aloud several times and explain what it means *aloud* (so your ears and brain can hear what you learned). Use the pronunciation key to help you practice if you are unsure.

adenectomy (ad ə nek′ tō mē)
adenitis (ad ə nī′ tis)
adenoma (ad ə nō′ mä)
arthroplasty (ärth′ rō plas′ tē)
arthrotomy (ärth rot′ ō mē)
carcinoma (kär sin ō′ mä)
cephalalgia (sef ə lal′ jē ä)
cephalic (se fal′ ik)
chondritis (kon drī′ tis)
colostomy (kō los′ tō mē)
dentalgia (den tal′ jē ä)
encephalitis (en sef ə lī′ tis)
encephalocele (en sef′ ə lō sēl)
encephaloma (en sef′ ə lō′ mä)
endosteoma (en dos tē ō′ mä)
exogenous (eks oj′ ə nus)
histology (his tol′ ō jē)
hyperemesis (hī per em′ ə sis)
hypertrophy (hī per′ tro fē)
hypodermic (hī pō der′ mik)
intercostal (in ter kos′ t’l)
laryngitis (lair an jī′ tis)
lipoid (lip′ oid)
lipoma (lī pō′ mä)
morphology (mor fäl′ ō jē)
mucoid (myoo′ koid)
oncology (on kol′ ō jē)
osteitis (os tē ī′ tis)
osteomalacia (os′ tē ō mä lā′ zhə)
pathologist (path ol′ ō jist)
thyroidectomy (thī roy dek′ tō mē)
tracheotomy (trā kē ot′ ō mē)

Take a short break and then test yourself with the Chapter 2 Self-Test, next page.

Chapter 2 Self-Test

Part 1

From the list on the right, select the correct meaning for each of the terms in the left-hand column. Write the letters in the space provided.

______	1. Osteomalacia	a.	Overdevelopment
______	2. Intercostal	b.	Study of microscopic tissues
______	3. Emesis	c.	Surgical removal of cartilage
______	4. Adenoma	d.	Between the ribs
______	5. Laryngotomy	e.	Surgical repair of a joint
______	6. Lipoid	f.	Softening of bone tissue
______	7. Cephalalgia	g.	Herniation of brain tissue
______	8. Morphology	h.	Tumor of glandular tissue
______	9. Carcinogenic	i.	Headache
______	10. Encephalocele	j.	Incision into the larynx
______	11. Arthroplasty	k.	Pertainiing to producing cancer
______	12. Oncologist	l.	Resembling fat
______	13. Hypertrophy	m.	Vomiting, to vomit
______	14. Chondrectomy	n.	Medical specialist dealing with tumors
______	15. Histology	o.	The science of studying the structure of an organ

Part 2

Complete each of the medical terms on the right with the appropriate prefix and/or suffix:

1. Surgical removal of the thyroid gland	Thyroid ____________
2. Inflammation of glandular tissue	Aden ____________
3. Malignant tumor	Carcin ____________
4. Excessive vomiting	____________ emesis
5. Resembling mucus	Muc ____________
6. Tumor specialist	Onc ____________
7. Making a new permanent opening into the colon	Col ____________
8. Inflammation inside the head	______ cephal ______
9. Tumor of fat tissue	____________ oma
10. Pertaining to the teeth	Dent ____________
11. To breathe out	____________ hale
12. Pertaining to between the ribs	______ cost ______
13. A tumor inside the bone canal	______ oste ______
14. Medical condition resulting from an *under*active thyroid	______ thyroid ______
15. Originating or produced completely outside of an organ or organism	____________ genous

ANSWERS

Part 1	*Part 2*
1. f.	1. Thyroidectomy
2. d.	2. Adenitis
3. m.	3. Carcinoma
4. h.	4. Hyperemesis
5. j.	5. Mucoid
6. l.	6. Oncologist
7. i.	7. Colostomy
8. o.	8. Encephalitis
9. k.	9. Lipoma

10. g.	10. Dental
11. e.	11. Exhale
12. n.	12. Intercostal
13. a.	13. Endosteoma
14. c.	14. Hypothyroidism
15. b.	15. Exogenous

3 Basic Anatomical Terms and Abnormal Conditions

In Chapter 3 you will put together 40 new medical terms. You'll work with some new prefixes and suffixes and practice using those you covered in earlier chapters. Although this program doesn't attempt to teach anatomy of the human body, the language of medicine is all about the human body and what affects its parts. So in this chapter you'll bring anatomy and medicine together by focusing on a couple of anatomical areas and some abnormal conditions that affect them.

In Chapter 3 and beyond you will find that terms are largely grouped by body system: for example, terms dealing with the heart are grouped together, and terms dealing with the gastrointestinal system are grouped together. Further, we will discuss why most medical practitioners use these groupings as an important tool of communication.

Mini-Glossary

Root Words

abdomin/o (*abdomen*)
cephal/o (*head*)
chol/e (*bile, gall*)
cocc/i (*coccus*)
crani/o (*cranium, skull*)
cyst/o (*bladder, sac*)
dipl/o (*double*)
hydro (*water*)
lith/o (*stone, calculus*)
metr/o, meter (*measure*)
ot/o (*ear*)
pelv/i (*pelvis*)
phob/ia (*fear*)
py/o (*pus*)
rhin/o (*nose*)
staphyl/o (*grape*)
strept/o (*chain*)
therap/o (*treatment*)
thorac/o (*thorax*)

Prefixes	**Suffixes**
ab- (*away from*)	-ar (*pertaining to*)
ad- (*toward*)	-centesis (*puncture* of a cavity)
	-genesis, gen/o (*produce, originate*)
	-meter (*measuring instrument*)
	-orrhea (*flow, discharge*)

Before you begin Chapter 3, take the time to complete the Review Sheet for Chapter 2. It will refresh your memory of the terms and word parts you studied. It may surprise you to find out how much you've learned. Try it (page 263).

1.
The prefix *ab*- means from or away from.
Abnormal means ____________________ normal.

away from

2.
The prefix ab- means ____________________.

from or away from

3.
Ab/errant uses the prefix ab- before the English word for wandering. What do you think the term ab/errant means? ____________________
____

wandering from (the normal course of events)

4.
Ab/errant is used in medicine to describe a structure that wanders from the normal. When some nerve fibers follow an unusual route, they form an ________ / ________________ nerve.

ab/errant
aberrant
ab er′ ant

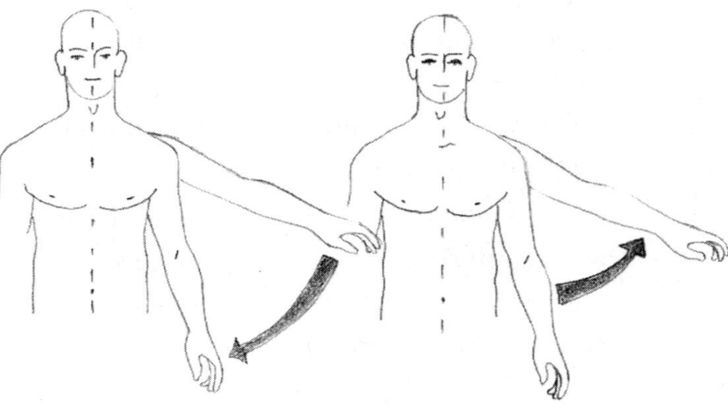

Figure 3.1 Adduction/Abduction

aberrant

5.
Aberrant nerves wander from the normal nerve track. Blood vessels that follow an unusual path are called ________________ vessels.

ab/duction
abduction
ab duk′ shun

6.
Ab/duct/ion means movement away from a midline. When the arm is raised from the side of the body,
________ / ____________________ has occurred.
away from (midline) — movement

abducted

7.
When children have been kidnapped and taken from their parents, they have been ________________.

abducted

8.
Abduction can occur from any midline. When the fingers of the hand are spread apart, four fingers have been ________________ from the midline of the hand.

ad/duction
adduction
ad duk′ shun

9.
On the other hand, *ad-* is a prefix meaning toward. Movement toward a midline is ________ / ________________.

ab-
ad-

10.
The prefix meaning from or away from is ________. The prefix meaning toward, or toward the midline, is ________.

ad/<u>hesion</u>

11.
When two normally separate tissues join together, they adhere to each other like adhesive tape. Underline the part of the word that means sticking or joining: ad/hesion.

ad/hesion
adhesion
ad hē′ zhun

12.
Several years ago patients did not walk quickly after surgery, which sometimes resulted in abnormal joining of tissues to each other as an adverse effect. Write the word that means the abnormal joining and healing together of tissues: ________ / ________________.

adhesions

13.
Now patients walk the day following an appendectomy. This has nearly eliminated ________________.

14.

Here's a quick review exercise.

Complete the following:

away from	The prefix ab- means __________________ the midline.
toward	The prefix ad- means __________________ the midline.

In your own words, explain the meaning of the following terms:

movement away from the midline	abduction __________________
sticking or joining together	adhesion __________________
a structure that wanders from the normal	aberrant __________________
a condition away from normal	abnormal __________________
movement toward a midline	adduction __________________

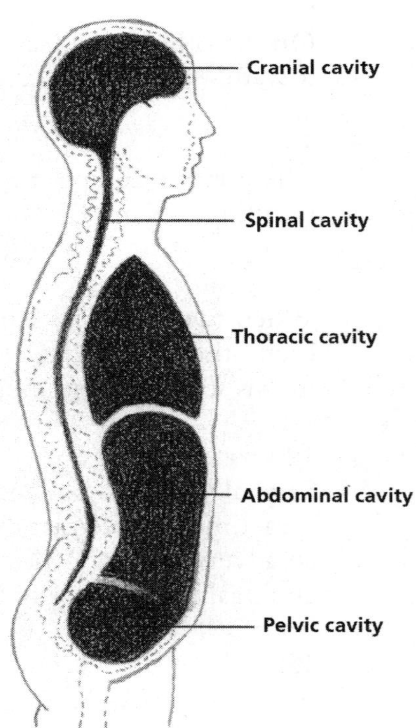

Figure 3.2 The Great Cavities

The great cavities are closed cavities not open to the outside of the body. Many of the body organs are suspended in these internal chambers and provide cushions against shocks. The cavities allow body organs to assume various sizes and shapes. The *cranial cavity* and *spinal cavity* are continuous and house the brain and spinal cord. The *thoracic cavity* contains the lungs and major blood vessels and other structures. The *abdominal cavity* is where the stomach, liver, spleen, and intestines are found. The lower portion of the abdominal cavity is set apart as the *pelvic cavity*. Here's where the female reproductive organs, urinary bladder, and male ducts may be found.

cranium (crani/o)	thorax (thorac/o)
abdomen (abdomino/o)	pelvis (pelv/i)

Refer to Figure 3.2 to help you complete many of the following frames.

belly, abdominal cavity, or abdomen
ab dō′ men
of or pertaining to the abdomen, or abdominal cavity

15.
Abdomin/o is used to form words about the abdominal cavity or belly. When you see abdomin/o in a word, you think of the ____________________.

Abdomin/al is an adjective that means ____________________________ ____.

abdomin/o/centesis
abdominocentesis
ab dom′ i nō sen tē′ sis

16.
Abdomin/o/centesis means puncturing the abdominal cavity to remove fluid. This is a surgical puncture of a cavity. The word for surgical puncture of the abdominal cavity is ____________________ / ______ / ______________________.
abdomen　　puncture of a cavity

abdominocentesis

17.
Centesis, or surgical puncture of a cavity, is a word in itself. Build a term meaning surgical puncture or tapping of the abdomen: ____________________________.

abdominocentesis

18.
When fluid has accumulated in the abdominal cavity, it can be drained off by a procedure called ____________________________.

cardi/o/centesis
cardiocentesis
kär′ dē ō sen tē′ sis

19.
Try this. The word for surgical puncture of a heart chamber is ________________ / ______ / ______________________.
heart　　puncture of a cavity

20.

cyst

Abdomin/o/cyst/ic means pertaining to the abdomen and urinary bladder. The word root for bladder is __________.

bladder

Cyst/o is used to form terms that refer to the ______________.

cyst/o

To refer to the urinary bladder or any sac containing fluid, use some form of __________ / _____.

21.

cyst/otomy
cystotomy

The word for temporary incision into a bladder is __________ / ______________.
bladder / incision into (temporary)

cyst/itis
cystitis

Inflammation of a bladder is ______________.

cyst/ectomy
cystectomy

The word for surgical removal of a bladder is ______________.

22.

Chances are good that by now you have figured out how word parts go together to create meaning. But let's review a simple rule and some examples.

Rule: About 90 percent of the time, the meaning of a term can be unscrambled by identifying its component parts in reverse.

For example,
cyst means bladder;
-itis means inflammation of.

inflammation of the bladder

Therefore, cystitis means ______________________________.

Dermat means skin;
-ologist means a specialist (one who studies).

one who studies the skin, or a skin specialist

Therefore, dermatologist means ______________________________.

Abdomino means abdomen;
-centesis means surgical puncture of a cavity (to drain off fluid).

puncture of the abdominal cavity (to drain fluid)

Therefore, abdominocentesis means ______________________________.

	23. Take a look at Figure 3.2.
pertaining to the abdomen and thorax (bony cage forming the chest cavity)	The bony cage that forms the chest cavity is called the *thorax*. What does abdomin/o/thorac/ic mean? ______________________________ ______________________________
abdomin/o/thorac/ic abdominothoracic ab dom′ ə nō thō rā′ sik	24. A word that means, literally, pertaining to the abdomen and chest cavity is ________ / ____ / ________ / ______. (abdomen) (thorax) (pertaining to)
thorac/ic thoracic thō rā′ sik	25. *Thorac/o* forms words about the thorax, or chest cavity. A word that means pertaining to the chest cavity is ________ / ______. (thorax) (pertaining to)
thorac/otomy thoracotomy thōr ə kot′ ə mē	26. Write a term meaning incision into the chest cavity: ________ / ________.
thorac/o/centesis thoracocentesis thōr′ ə kō sen tē′ sis	27. Write a term meaning surgical puncturing of the chest cavity to remove fluids: ________ / ____ / ________. (thorax) (puncture of)
thorac/o/plast/y thoracoplasty thōr′ ə kō plas′ tē	28. A word for the surgical repair of the chest cage is ________ / ____ / plast / y.
cyst/o/plast/y cystoplasty sis′ tō plas′ tē	29. Now write a word for surgical repair of a bladder: ________ / ____ / ________ / ____.
water, fluid, or a watery fluid	30. A hydro/cyst is a sac (or bladder) filled with watery fluid. *Hydro* is used in words to mean ______________________________ ______________.

31.
Go back to Figure 3.2. The space inside the head is called ______________________________.

the cranial cavity

Cranium means skull. Cephal/o is the combining form meaning ______________________________.

head, including cranium and facial bones

Therefore, cephalic means ______________________________.

of or pertaining to the head

32.
An increased amount of fluid in the head is called hydro/cephal/us. Both the fluid and the brain occupy the same space, called the ______________________________.

cranial cavity

33.
A disease characterized by an enlarged head due to an increased amount of fluid in the cranial cavity is called ______________ / ______________ / us.
(water) (head)

hydro/cephal/us
hydrocephalus
hī′ drō sə fal′ us

34.
Unless resolved, accumulation of watery fluid in the cranial cavity results in deformity of the skull, and brain damage may occur. This condition is called ______________________.

hydrocephalus

35.
Hydro/phob/ia means having an abnormal fear of water. *Phobia* means ______________________.

abnormal fear

36.
An abnormal fear of water is ______________ / ______________ / __________.
(water) (abnormal fear)

hydro/phob/ia
hydrophobia
hī drō fō′ bē ə

37.
Therapy means treatment. Treatment by means of water is ______________ / ______________.
(water) (treatment)

hydro/therapy
hydrotherapy
hī′ drō ther′ ə pē

Swirling water baths are a form of ______________________.

hydrotherapy

38.
See Figure 3.2 again. The bones of the pelvis form the pelvic cavity. A physician measures the size of a woman's pelvic cavity after she becomes pregnant. This procedure is called pelvi/metr/y.

pelvi — The word root for pelvic cavity is ______________.

metr — The root for measurement is ______________.

-y — The ending meaning a procedure is ___________.

39.
pelvimetry
pel vim′ ə trē

To determine whether a woman has a pelvis large enough to avoid trouble during labor, a physician can measure the size of the pelvic cavity. This measurement is called ________________.

40.
a measuring device used for pelvimetry (or equivalent)

What do you think a pelvimeter is? ______________________________
____
____

41.
pelvimetry
pelvimeter
pel vim′ ə ter

When a physician measures the patient's pelvic cavity, the doctor is making a measurement called ________________.

The instrument used is a ________________.

42.
surgical repair of the skull or cranium

Crani/o is used in terms referring to the cranial cavity or crani/um, or skull. Crani/o/plast/y means ____________________________
____.

43.
Write a medical term for each of the following:

crani/ectomy
craniectomy
krā nē ek′ tō mē

a surgical procedure to excise part of the cranium
______________ / ________________
skull — excision of

crani/otomy
craniotomy
krā nē ot′ ō mē

incision into the skull
______________ / ______________
cranium — incision into

crani/o/meter
craniometer

an instrument to measure the cranium
______________ / _____ / ______________

44.
The cerebrum occupies the cranial cavity. Thinking occurs in the cerebrum (cerebr/o). What is the meaning of crani/o/cerebr/al?

____

____

of, or pertaining to, the brain and skull (cranium)

45.
Have you ever been told to use your "gray matter"? Gray matter controls thinking, feeling, and movement. The gray matter is the largest part of the brain. What is it called? ______________ (cranium or cerebrum)

cerebrum

46.
Write a term meaning of, or pertaining to, the gray matter of the brain: ______________ (cerebrum) / ________ (pertaining to).

cerebr/al
cerebral
ser ē′ brəl

47.
Cerebr/o/spin/al refers to the brain and spinal cord. What part of the word means pertaining to the spinal cord?
______________ / ________

spin/al
spinal
spī′ nəl

48.
A puncture or tap to remove fluid from the space around the cerebrum and spinal cord is called a spinal tap or
______________ (cerebrum) / _____ / ______________ (spinal) / ________ (pertaining to) puncture.

cerebr/o/spin/al
cerebrospinal
ser ē brō spī′ nvl

49.
Here's a quick review exercise.

SUGGESTED ANSWERS:

head	pelvis
bladder, sac	bony vault, skull
abdomen	chest cavity, rib cage
measurement	water, fluid

Using the suggested answers (only if you must), write the meaning of each of the following:

pelv/i ______________________________
hydro- ______________________________
cyst/o ______________________________
cephal/o ______________________________

pelvis, pelvic cavity
water, fluid
bladder, sac
head

measurement, meter — metr/o ________________
bony chest cage, thorax — thorac/o ________________
bony vault (brain), skull — crani/o ________________
abdomen, abdominal cavity — abdomin/o ________________

50.
Try that again.

SUGGESTED ANSWERS:

-therapy	-otomy
-plasty	-metry
-ectomy	-centesis

Some suggestions: (Yours may be different.)

Add a prefix or ending to each of the following combining forms and then explain the meaning of the term you created.

crani/o ________________
____

craniotomy

pelv/i ________________
____

pelvimetry

thorac/o ________________
____

thoracoplasty

abdomin/o ________________
____

abdominocentesis

cyst/o ________________
____

cystectomy

hydro- ________________
____

hydrotherapy

51.
Let's try something different. Coccus is a bacteria that causes disease. Cocc/i is the plural of cocc/us. When building terms about a whole family of bacteria called the cocci, we use the word root ________.

cocc-

(See Appendix B for more information on the formation of plurals.)

52.
Pneumonia is caused by the pneumococcus. From this term you know that the germ responsible for pneumonia belongs to the family of bacteria called ________ / ____ (plural).

cocc/i
kok′ sē

53.
There are three main types of a coccus bacteria:

	cocci growing in pairs are
dipl/o/cocc/i	dipl / o / ____________ / _____,
	cocci growing in twisted chains are
strept/o/cocc/i	strept / o / ____________ / _____,
	cocci growing in clusters are
staphyl/o/cocc/i	staphyl / o / ____________ / _____.

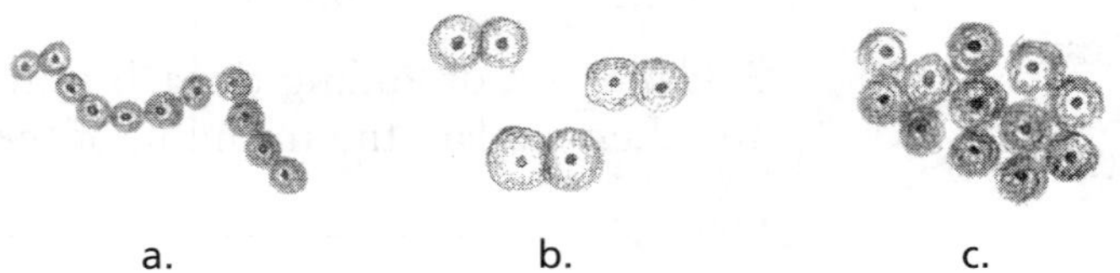

Figure 3.3 Cocci Bacteria

(a. strept) (b. diplo) (c. staphyl)

Bacteria (pl.) of the coccus family are round or spheroidal shaped single-cell micro-organisms. Many types of cocci (pl.) exist and cause illness and infection in humans.

54.
Refer to the illustration above for help. If you see a twisted chain of cocci when examining a slide under a microscope, you would say they were ______________ / _____ / ____________ / _____.

strept/o/cocc/i
strep′ tō kok sē

55.
Staphyle is the Greek word for bunch of grapes. If you should see a cluster of cocci when using a microscope, you would say they were ____________________ / _____ / ____________ / _____.

staphyl/o/cocc/i
staphylococci
staf′ i lō kok′ sī

56.
The bacteria that cause carbuncles grow in clusters like bunches of grapes. Carbuncles are caused by ___________________ bacteria.

staphylococci

pertaining to producing pus

57.
Py/o is used for words involving pus. Genesis (gen/o) is from a Greek word meaning produce or originate. Py/o/gen/ic means ______________________.

py/o/gen/ic
pyogenic

58.
Staphylococci produce pus; therefore, these cocci are ______ / ____ / ________ / ______ bacteria.
pus producing

pyogenic

59.
Bacteria that contain or produce pus are referred to as ______________________ bacteria.

pyogenic

60.
Boils are purulent (contain pus). This pus is formed by ______________ bacteria.
pus-producing

discharge of pus

61.
The suffix *-orrhea* means flow or discharge. Py/orrhea means ______________________________.

py/orrhea
pyorrhea
pī ō rē′ ə

62.
The suffix -orrhea refers to any flow or discharge. A flow of pus is called ______ / ____________.
pus discharge

pyorrhea

63.
Pyorrhea alveolaris is a disease of the teeth and gums. The term that tells you pus is being discharged is ____________.

pyorrhea

64.
When pus flows from the salivary gland, the disease is called ______________ salivaris (of the salivary gland).

ear

65.
Ot/orrhea means a discharging ear; *ot-* is the word root for ____.

ot/orrhea
otorrhea
ō tō rē′ ə

66.
Ot/orrhea is both a symptom and a disease. No matter which is meant, the word to use is ______ / ____________.
ear discharge

67.
Otorrhea may be a sign of ot/itis media (middle). Ot/itis media means ______________________________.

inflammation of the (middle) ear

This disease involves discharge, inflammation, pain, and deafness. What's the term for discharge from the ear? ______________

otorrhea

68.
Otitis usually causes ear pain. Write the medical term for ear pain: ________ / ____________.
(ear) (pain)

ot/algia
otalgia

69.
Small children often complain of an earache. The medical term for pain in the ear is ______________.

otalgia
ō tal′ jē ə

70.
Rhinorrhea means discharge from the nose. *Rhin/o* is used in terms about the ____________.

nose

71.
Taking what is necessary from rhin/o, form a term meaning inflammation of the nose: __________ / __________.

rhin/itis
rhinitis
rī nī′ tis

72.
When your head cold is accompanied by a "runny nose" the medical term for the symptom is __________ / ______________.
(nose) (discharge)

rhin/orrhea
rhinorrhea

73.
Irritated or diseased sinuses in the head and face may discharge fluid through the nose. This is a form of ______________.

rhinorrhea

74.
Build a term that means surgical repair of the nose: __________ / _____ / ____________.

rhin/o/plasty
rhinoplasty

Form a word that means incision into the nose: ________________ / __________________.

rhin/otomy
rhinotomy

75.
Try these for a quick review.

SUGGESTED ANSWERS:

twisted, chainlike	double, paired
family of bacteria	producing, originating
pus	grapelike cluster
ear	nose

Using the suggestsions above (only if you must), write the meaning of each of the following:

Answer	
family of bacteria	cocc/us, cocc/i ______
grapelike cluster	staphyl/o ______
pus	py/o ______
nose	rhin/o ______
double, paired	dipl/o ______
ear	ot/o ______
twisted, chainlike	strept/o ______
producing, originating	gen/o ______

76.
Try again. Here are some word parts and combining forms to help you build some familiar medical terms.

rhin/o	cocc/i
ot/o	py/o
-plasty	-orrhea
staphyl/o	gen/o
-algia	dipl/o

Put together a medical term that best defines each of the following descriptions:

Answer	
diplococci	A family of coccus bacteria found growing in pairs ______
pyogenic	Pertaining to producing pus, or pus-forming ______
rhinorrhea	A runny discharge from the nose ______
otalgia	Pain in the ear, earache ______
staphylococci	Bacteria of the coccus family growing in grapelike clusters ______
rhinoplasty	Surgical repair (reconstruction) of the nose ______

77.
A rhin/o/lith is a calculus or stone in the nose. *Lith/o* is the combining form for ________________.

Answer: calculus or stone

78.
Lithogenesis means producing or forming ________________.

Answer: calculi (plural of calculus) or stones

79.
Taking what is necessary from lith/o, build a word meaning an incision for the removal of a stone:
____________ / ____________.
stone / incision into (for)

Answer: lith/otomy
lithotomy
lith ot′ə mē

80.
Calculi or stones form in many places in the body. A chol/e/lith is a gallstone. Chole is the word for ________________.

Answer: gall or bile

81.
One cause of gallbladder disease is the presence of a gallstone or
____________ / ____________.
gall / stone

Answer: chole/lith
cholelith

82.
No matter what its size or shape, irritation and blockage of the gallbladder can be caused by a bile or gallstone, called ____________.

Answer: cholelith

83.
Gall is the fluid stored in the gallbladder. Cholecyst is a medical name for the ________________.

Answer: gallbladder

84.
When gallstones cause inflammation of the gallbladder, this condition is called
____________ / ____________ / ____________.
gall / bladder / inflammation

Answer: chole/cyst/itis
cholecystitis
kō′ lē sis tī′ tis

85.
Inflammation of the gallbladder is accompanied by pain and emesis. The condition is called ________________.

Answer: cholecystitis

86.
Fatty foods like butter, cream, and whole milk contain fat and can exacerbate inflammation in the gallbladder. These foods should be avoided by patients with an inflammatory condition of the gallbladder, or ________________.

Answer: cholecystitis

chole/cyst/otomy
cholecystotomy
kō lē sis tot′ e mē
or
chole/lith/otomy
cholelithotomy
kō′ lē lith ot′ ə mē

87.
When a cholelith causes cholecystitis, one of two surgical procedures may solve the problem. One is an incision into the gallbladder to remove stones, called a
__________ / __________ / __________
gall stone incision into
or __________ / __________ / __________.
gall stone incision into

chole/cyst/ectomy
cholecystectomy
kō′ lē sis tek′ tō mē

88.
More often, the presence of a gallstone calls for excision of the gallbladder, called
__________ / __________ / __________.
gall bladder surgical removal

89.
It's time to review. From List B select the best meaning for each term in List A. Write your choice in the space provided.

Answer	LIST A		LIST B
pelvis	pelv/i	__________	measure
stone, calculus	lith/o	__________	skull
gall, bile	chol/e	__________	pus
pus	py/o	__________	pelvis
skull	crani/o	__________	head
head	cephal/o	__________	gall, bile
measure	metr/o	__________	stone, calculus
nose	rhin/o	__________	chainlike
ear	ot/o	__________	double, pairs
chainlike	strept/o	__________	chest, thorax
grapelike	staphyl/o	__________	bladder, sac
double	dipl/o	__________	nose
chest	thorac/o	__________	abdomen
bladder, sac	cyst/o	__________	grapelike
abdomen	abdomin/o	__________	ear

90.
Complete the following:

away from — The prefix ab- means __________ the midline.

toward — The prefix ad- means __________ the midline.

watery fluid, water — The prefix hydro- means __________.

Answers	91. Select the best meaning for each of the following word parts.	
treatment	therapy ______________	surgical puncture
calculus, stone	lith ______________	abnormal fear
discharge, flow	orrhea ______________	calculus, stone
surgical puncture	centesis ______________	treatment
abnormal fear	phobia ______________	discharge, flow

92.

Each of the suffixes below means *of,* or *pertaining to* the word root to which it is attached. Write the meaning of each term.

Answers	SUFFIXES	EXAMPLE	MEANING
of or pertaining to the duodenum	-al	duoden/al	______________
pertaining to the stomach	-ic	gastr/ic	______________
pertaining to the lumbar area (of the spine)	-ar	lumb/ar	______________
pertaining to the heart	-ac	cardi/ac	______________

93.

Here are 40 new medical terms you formed in Chapter 3. Read them one at a time and pronounce each aloud. Better yet, ask a friend to say them aloud and you spell them.

aberrant (ab er′ ant)
abdominal (ab dom′ i nəl)
abdominocentesis (ab dom′ i nō sen tē′ sis)
abduction (ab duk′ shun)
adduction (ad duk′ shun)
cardiocentesis (kär′ dē ō sen tē′sis)
cephalic (cə fal′ ik)
cholecystectomy (kō′ lē sis tek′ tō mē)
cholecystitis (kō′ lē sis tī′ tis)
cholelithotomy (kō′ lē lith ot′ ə mē)
craniectomy (krā nē ek′ tō mē)
cranioplasty (krā′ nē ō plas′ tē)
craniotomy (krā nē ot′ ō mē)
cranium (krā′ nē um)
cystitis (sis tī′ tis)
cystocele (sis′ to sēl)
cystotomy (sis tot′ ə mē)
diplococci (dip′ lō kok′ sī)
hydrocephalus (hī′ drō sə fal′ us)
hydrophobia (hī′ drō fō′ bē ə)
hydrotherapy (hī′ drō ther′ ə pē)
lithogenesis (lith′ ō jen′ ə sis)
lithotomy (lith ot′ ō mē)
otalgia (ō tal′ jē a)
otitis (ō tī′ tis)
otorrhea (ō tō rē′ ə)
pelvic (pel′ vik)
pelvimetry (pel vim′ ə trē)

pyogenic (pī ō jen′ ik)
pyorrhea (pī ō rē′ ə)
rhinitis (rī nī′ tis)
rhinolith (rī′ nō lith)
rhinoplasty (rī′ nō plas tē)
rhinorrhea (rī nōr rē′ ə)
staphylococci (staf′ i lō kok′ sī)
streptococci (strep′ tō kok′ sī)
thoracic (thō rā′ sik)
thoracocentesis (thōr′ ə kō sen tē′ sis)
thoracoplasty (thōr′ ə kō plas′ tē)
thoracotomy (thōr ə kot′ ə mē)

Take the Chapter 1 Self-Test before going on.

Chapter 3 Self-Test

Part 1

From the list on the right, select the correct meaning for each of the following terms. Write the letter in the space provided.

______ 1. Thoracocentesis
______ 2. Cholelithotomy
______ 3. Otorrhea
______ 4. Cystotomy
______ 5. Abdominalgia
______ 6. Cranium
______ 7. Cephalgia
______ 8. Hydrophobia
______ 9. Adduction
______ 10. Streptococci
______ 11. Pyogenic
______ 12. Aberrant
______ 13. Pelvic
______ 14. Cholecystotomy
______ 15. Rhinoplasty

a. Headache
b. Relating to the pelvis, pelvic cavity
c. Wandering or out of the normal place
d. Tapping or puncturing the chest cavity (thorax) to remove fluid
e. Movement toward the midline
f. Abnormal fear of water
g. Running or draining from the ear
h. Incision into the bladder
i. Producing pus
j. The bony vault surrounding the brain
k. Incision for the purpose of removing a gallstone
l. Commonly referred to as a "bellyache"
m. Cocci bacteria that grow in chains
n. Surgical repair or restoration of the nose
o. Incision into the gallbladder

Part 2

Complete each of the medical terms on the right with the appropriate word root:

1. Herniation of a bladder ________________ cele
2. Tapping or puncturing of the heart chamber ________________ centesis
3. Surgical repair of the bony vault that encloses the brain ________________ plasty
4. Earache ________________ algia
5. Gallstone ________________ lith
6. Inflammation of the nose ________________ itis
7. Measurement of the pelvis ________________ metry
8. Relating to the thorax ________________ ic
9. Collection of fluid in the head Hydro ________________
10. Incision into the cranium ________________ otomy
11. Relating to the formation of pus ________________ genic
12. Surgical repair of the chest cage ________________ plasty
13. Instrument for measuring the pelvis ________________ meter
14. Relating to the abdomen ________________ al
15. Surgical removal of the gallbladder ________________

ANSWERS

Part 1	***Part 2***
1. d	1. Cystocele
2. k	2. Cardiocentesis
3. g	3. Cranioplasty
4. h	4. Otalgia
5. l	5. Cholelith
6. j	6. Rhinitis
7. a	7. Pelvimetry
8. f	8. Thoracic
9. e	9. Hydrocephalus

10. m	10. Craniotomy
11. i	11. Pyogenic
12. c	12. Thoracoplasty
13. b	13. Pelvimeter
14. o	14. Abdominal
15. n	15. Cholecystectomy

4 The Genitals and the Urinary Tract

Chapter 4 addresses the genitourinary system. As the name suggests, this system includes the genitals and the urinary system. This section of the head-to-toe assessment is documented differently depending on the sex of the client, and you will find many of the medical terms subdivided in the book. This section provides information on urinary patterns, obstructions (blockages), and problems. This includes information about the bladder—the organ that stores urine—and the tubes that lead to and from the bladder to remove urine from the body. It also has information involving reproduction, fertility, and sexuality, and addresses any relevant problems that might arise. Review the mini-glossary below.

Chapter 4 is a little longer than the previous ones. Again, you'll be working with roots, prefixes, and suffixes. You'll make about 50 new medical terms and practice defining them. You'll work with anatomical terms and some medical conditions associated with these areas of the body. There are illustrations showing the anatomy of the urinary tract and the genital organs of both male and female. Make these illustrations work for you. Bookmark the pages and refer to them often. Move slowly. When you encounter a difficult example, go back a frame or two and work through it again. Help yourself understand before moving on.

Mini-Glossary

Root Words

angi/o (*vessel*)
arter/i/o (*artery*)
blast/o (*embryo*)
colp/o (*vagina*)
crypt/o (*hidden*)
fibr/o (*fiber*)
hem/o, hemat/o (*blood*)
hyster/o (*uterus*)
kinesi/o (*motion*)
lys/o (*destruction*)

men/o (*menses*)
my/o (*muscle*)
nephr/o (*kidney*)
neur/o (*nerve*)
o/o (*egg, ovum*)
oophor/o (*ovary*)
orchid/o (*testes*)
peps/o, peps/ia (*digestion*)
pyel/o (*pelvis of the kidney*)
salping/o (*fallopian tube*)
scler/o (*tough, hard*)
spermat/o (*sperm*)
ureter/o (*ureter*)
urethr/o (*urethra*)
ur/o (*urine*)

Prefixes

a-, an- (*without*)
dys- (*pain*)

Suffixes

-blast (*embryonic*)
-y, -ia (*noun ending*)
-orrhagia (*hemorrhage*)
-orrhaphy (*suture*)
-pexy (*fixation*)
-ptosis (*drooping*)
-spasm (*twitching*)
-sperm (*sperm*)

Did you remember to complete the Chapter 3 Review Sheet before beginning this new unit? Practice, practice, practice. It really works (page 265).

pain on movement or movement pain

1.
Kinesi is used in words to mean movement or motion. Kinesi/algia means ____.

kinesi/algia
kinesialgia
kin ē′ sē al′ jē ə

2.
When moving any sore or injured part of the body, pain occurs. Moving a broken arm can cause pain described as ______________ / ______________.

kinesialgia

3.
After your first horseback ride, almost any movement causes a condition called ______________.

Answer	Frame
kinesi/ology kinesiology kin ē′ sē ol′ ə jē	4. The suffix *-ology* means study of. (Remember -ologist?) The study of muscular movements is __________ / __________. movement / study of
kinesiology	5. Kinesi/ology is the study of movement. The study of muscular movement during exercise is known as the scientific field of __________.
kinesiology	6. The whole science of how the body moves is embraced in the field of __________.
dys-	7. The prefix *dys-* means painful, bad, or difficult. Dys/men/orrhea means painful menstruation. The prefix for painful, bad, or difficult is ______.
poor or painful digestion	8. *Pepsis* (peps/o) is the Greek word for digestion. Dys/peps/ia means ______________________________.
dys/peps/ia dyspepsia dis pep′ sē ə	9. Eating under tension may cause painful or poor digestion. This is called ________ / __________ / ______.
dyspepsia	10. Contemplating the troubles of the world while eating is a good way to cause __________.
	11. Here's a quick review of what you just covered. From List B select the best meaning for each term in List A. Write your choice in the space provided.

Answer	LIST A	LIST B
menses	men/o __________	digestion
digestion	peps/o __________	movement
movement	kinesi/o __________	menses
painful	dys- __________	painful
without, absence of	a- __________	without, absence of

Refer to the table below to work through the next thirteen frames.

Some Combining Forms	
angi/o	vessel, blood & lymphatic
arteri/o	artery
fibr/o	fibrous, fiber
hem/o, hemat/o	blood
malac/o	soft, softened
lip/o	fat
my/o	muscle
neur/o	nerve or neuron
scler/o	hard
Some Suffixes	
-lysis	declining, dissolution
-spasm	twitch, twitching
-blast	germ or immature
-osis	condition of
-oma	tumor
-ia, -y	these endings make the term a noun

12.

neur/o/blast
neuroblast
nyo͞o′ ro blast

An immature (germ) cell from which muscle tissue develops is a my/o/blast. A germ cell from which a nerve cell develops is a ____________ / _____ / ______________.

13.

angi/o/blast
angioblast
an′ jē ō blast

A germ cell from which vessels develop is an ____________ / _____ / ______________.

14.

A spasm of a nerve is a neur/o/spasm.

my/o/spasm
myospasm
mī′ ō spa zm

A spasm of a muscle is a ________ / _____ / ______________.

angi/o/spasm
angiospasm
an′ jē ō spa′ zm

A spasm of a vessel is an ____________ / _____ / ______________.

15.

angi/o/scler/osis
angiosclerosis
an′ jē ō sklə rō′ sis

A (condition of) hardening of nerve tissue is neur/o/scler/osis. A hardening of a vessel is ____________ / _____ / ______________ / ____________.

vessel — hardening — condition of

my/o/scler/osis
myosclerosis
mī′ ō sklə rō′ sis

A hardening of muscle tissue is
_______ / _____ / ______________ / __________.

16.

neur/o/fibr/oma
neurofibroma
nyo͞o′ rō′ fī brō′ mä

angi/o/fibr/oma
angiofibroma
an′ jē ō fī brō′ mä

A tumor containing muscle and fibrous connective tissue is a my/o/fibr/oma. A tumor containing fibrous connective tissue and nerve tissue is a
__________ / _____ / ______________ / __________.
nerve / fibrous tissue / tumor

A vessel tumor containing fibrous connective tissue is a(n)
__________ / _____ / ______________ / __________.

17.

neur/o/lys/is
neurolysis
nyo͞o rol′ ə sis

angi/o/lys/is
angiolysis
an jē ol′ i sis

The destruction of muscle tissue is my/o/lys/is.

The destruction of nerve tissue is
__________ / _____ / __________ / _______.

The destruction or breaking down of vessels is
__________ / _____ / __________ / _______.

18.

arteri/o/scler/osis
arteriosclerosis
ar ter′ ē ō skler ō′ sis

Refer to the table only when you must. Arteri/o is used in words about the arteries. A word meaning hardening of the arteries is
____________ / _____ / ____________ / __________.

19.

arteri/o/scler/osis
arteriosclerosis

a softened artery
arteriomalacia
ar ter′ ē ō mä l1′ zha

Build a word meaning a hardened condition of the arteries:
____________ / _____ / ____________ / __________.

What do you think arteri/o/malac/ia means? ________________
____

20.

arteri/o/spasm
arteriospasm
ar ter′ ē ō spa′ zm

lip/o/lys/is
lipolysis
lip ol′ i sis

Build a word meaning arterial spasm:
____________ / _____ / __________.

Dissolution (breakdown) of fat is called
__________ / _____ / __________ / _____.

hem/angi/itis hemangiitis hē man′ jē ī tis hem/o/lysis hemolysis hē mol′ ə sis or another form is hemat/o/lysis hē mə tol′ ə sis	21. *Hem/o* refers to blood. A tumor of a blood vessel is a hem/angi/oma. (Note the dropped o.) An inflammation of a blood vessel is _______ / ________ / ________. Breaking down or dissolution of blood cells is _______ / ____ / ________.
hemat/o/logy hematology hē mə tol′ ə jē hemat/o/logist hematologist hē mə tol′ ə jist	22. Hemat/o also refers to blood. The study of blood is ________ / ____ / _______. One who specializes in the science of blood is a ________ / ____ / ___________.

23.

Let's go over the new material again briefly. Match the best definition in List B with the word root in List A. Write your selection in the space provided.

	LIST A	LIST B
artery	arteri/o ________________	fat
fibrous connective tissue	fibr/o ________________	muscle
blood	hem/o, hemat/o ________________	artery
fat	lip/o ________________	blood and lymph vessel
soften	malac/o ________________	soften
muscle	my/o ________________	harden
nerve	neur/o ________________	fibrous connective tissue
harden	scler/o ________________	blood
blood and lymph vessel	angi/o ________________	nerve

Now match the best definition in List B with the suffix in List A. Write the term.

	LIST A	LIST B
destruction of	-lysis ________________	tumor
twitching	-spasm ________________	science, or study of
tumor	-oma ________________	condition of
inflammation of	-itis ________________	twitching
germ cell (immature)	-blast ________________	inflammation of
condition of	-osis ________________	destruction of, dissolution
science, or study of	-ology ________________	germ cell (immature)

24.
Build a word for each of the following definitions.

Answer	Definition
	a condition of hardening of the arteries
arterio/scler/osis	______ / ______ / ______
hemat/oma	blood tumor ______ / ______
angio/spasm	blood vessel spasm ______ / ______
myo/fibr/oma or fibromyoma	fibrous muscle tumor ______ / ______ / ______
neuro/blast	nerve tissue germ cell ______ / ______
lipo/lysis	breakdown of fat tissue ______ / ______
dys/pepsia	poor or painful digestion ______ / ______

Take a break.

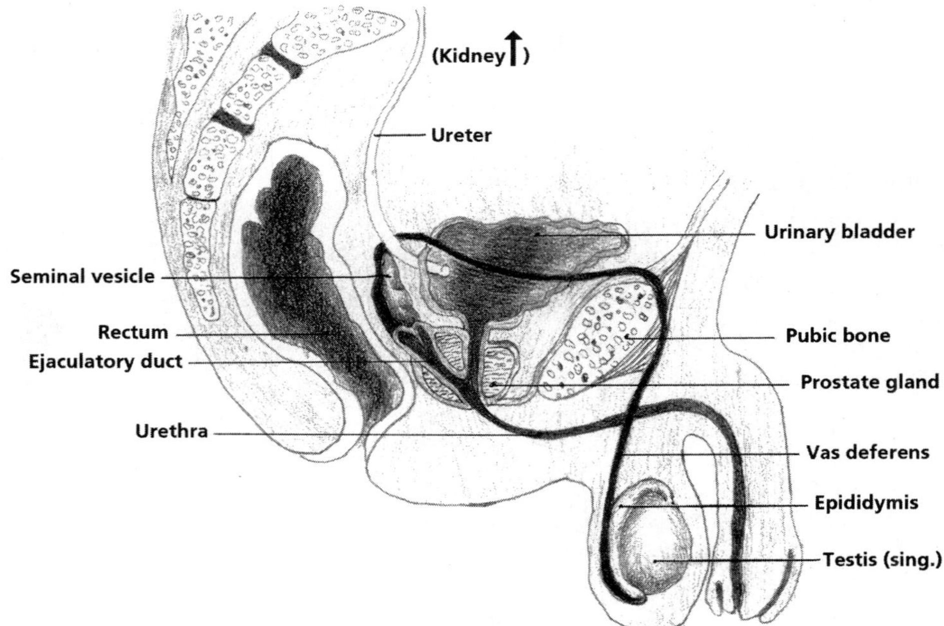

Figure 4.1 The Male Reproductive Organs (Midline Section)

The primary function of the male reproductive system is to produce *sperm cells* and deliver them to the female reproductive system for fertilization of the egg cells. The major organs of the male reproductive system are the paired *testes,* where sperm cells are produced. Surrounding the testis is a comma-shaped structure called the *epididymis*. Mature sperm cells are stored in the epididymis. The *vas deferens* is a long tube that conveys the mature sperm for ejaculation during copulation. It courses from the epididymis up into the body, over the pubic bone, curves to the left, passes the *urinary bladder,* curves again near the *ureter,* and passes downward. Here the vas joins with the duct leading from the *seminal vesicle* and forms the *ejaculatory duct*. The seminal vesicle is a small bladderlike structure that adds secretions to the sperm to form semen. The ejaculatory duct releases the semen and it enters the *urethra* as it exits the urinary bladder. The urethra is a 6- to 8-inch long tube in the male. It passes by the *prostate,* a chestnut-shaped gland surrounding the beginning of the urethra, and enters the penis, to deliver its contents for fertilization of the female egg cell.

Several accessory structures in the diagram show their relationships to the reproductive organs. The ureter can be seen near the urinary bladder. It delivers urine from the kidney. The last portion of the large intestine is the *rectum,* and the end of the digestive tract is the *anus.*

sperm or spermatazoon (spermat/o)
testis (orchid/o)
prostate (prostat-, prostat/o)
ureter (ureter/o)
urethra (urethr/o)

Review Figure 4.1, then refer to it as you work through frames 25 through 36.

25.
The testes are organs that manufacture sperm, the male germ cell; that is, spermatozoa (plural) are formed in the ________________.

testes (pl.)
testis (sing.)

26.
Orchid/algia means pain in a testicle or testis.

Orchid/ectomy means ________________________________
________________.

excision of a testicle, testis

27.
Build a word meaning

inflammation of a testicle ____________ / ________

orchid/itis
orchiditis
or ki dī′ tis

incision into a testis ____________ / _________

orchid/otomy
orchidotomy
or kid ot′ ō mē

28.
A crypt/ic remark is one with a hidden meaning. A crypt/ic belief is obscure. The word root for hidden or obscure is
________________.

crypt
kript′

29.
Near the time of birth the testes of the fetus normally descend from the abdominal cavity into the scrotum. Sometimes this fails to happen, and the testes are not evident at birth. This condition of undescended testes is called
___________ / ____________ / ism.
hidden testicle

crypt/orchid/ism
cryptorchidism
kript ôr′ kid ism

30.
When a testis is hidden in the abdominal cavity or is undescended, the condition is called ________________.

cryptorchidism

31.
An operation to repair cryptorchidism is called orchid/o/pexy. Circle the part of the term that means to fix in its place.

orchid/o/(pexy)

32.
Sperma is the Greek word meaning seed.
Spermat/o is used in words about spermat/o/zoa or male germ cells (sperm). Spermat/o/genesis means ______________________ ______________________.

formation of spermatozoa, sperm, or male germ cells

33.
Blast- means immature.
-lysis means dissolution or destruction.

Give a word meaning the destruction of spermatozoa:
____________ / ____ / ____________.

spermat/o/lysis
spermatolysis
sperm′ ə tol′ i sis

How about these:

an immature male cell, germ cell, sperm
____________ / ____ / ____________

spermat/o/blast
spermatoblast
sper mat′ ō blast

resembling sperm ____________ / ________

spermat/oid
spermatoid
sper′ mä toid

34.
Summarize what you learned:

my/o means ____________________.
angi/o means ____________________.
neur/o means ____________________.

muscle
vessel
nerve

35.
Again.

spasm means ______________________________.
blast/o means ______________________________.
scler/o means ______________________________.
fibr/o means ______________________________.
lysis means ______________________________.

twitching, spasm
germ cell (immature)
hard, hardened
fibrous
destruction of

36.
And these.

spermatozoa (sperm)	spermat/o means ______________________.
blood	hemat/o means ______________________.
blood	hem/o means ______________________.
formation of, or origination	genesis means ______________________.

Correct any definitions you may have missed; then cover the word roots, read the definitions you have written, and write the appropriate word root in the right-hand margin.

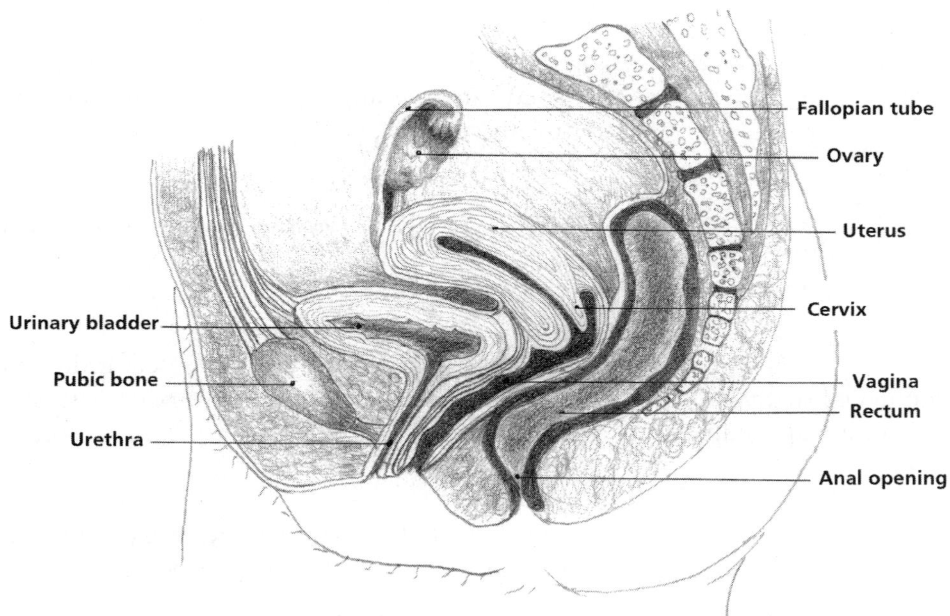

Figure 4.2 The Female Reproductive Organs (Midline Section)

The female reproductive system is responsible for producing female sex cells for potential union with male sperm cells. In addition, the female reproductive system nurtures the developing embryo and fetus for a nine-month period. The *ovaries* are the female reproductive organs in which egg cells are formed. An egg cell (*ovum*) is released into the *fallopian tube* and makes its way to the *uterus.* The uterus is a thick muscular organ that serves as a site for implantation of a fertilized ovum and nourishment of the embryo and fetus. A long narrow internal space leads from the uterus through a narrow neck called the *cervix*. The cervix is closed and passable only to microscopic entities unless a women is menstruating or in labor. The cervix opens into the vagina. The *vagina* is a tubular organ approximately four inches in length. It receives the semen from the penis and together with the cervix is the passageway to the uterus. It acts as a birth canal from the uterus to the outside for the newborn.

Other organs lie close to the female reproductive organs. Among these are the muscular *urinary bladder* and the *urethra*. The urethra is a short tube leading from the bladder that delivers urine to outside the body. The *rectum* is the last portion of the digestive organs and terminates at the *anus*.

ovary (oophor/o)	urinary bladder (cyst/o)
fallopian tube (salping/o)	urethra (urethr/o)
uterus (hyster/o)	vagina (colp/o)
ovum (o/o)	

Bookmark Figure 4.2 and refer to it as you work through frames 37 through 61.

37.
The Greek word for egg is *oon*. In scientific words, o/o (pronounce both o's) means egg or ovum. An o/o/blast is an immature ________________ cell.

egg (a cell that will become an ovum)

38.
An ovum is discharged from the ovary. The combining form used in words referring to the ovary is *oophor/o*.

What does oophor/ectomy mean? ________________

excision or surgical removal of the ovary

39.
Using what you need from oophor/o, build a word that means inflammation of an ovary: ________ / ________.

oophor/itis
oophoritis
ōō fôr ī′ tis

40.
Oophor- is the root for ovary. Build a term for each of the following:

excision of an ovary ________ / ________

tumor of an ovary (ovarian tumor)
________ / ________

oophor/ectomy
oophorectomy
ōō fôr ek′ tō mē

oophor/oma
oophoroma
ōō fôr ō′ ma

Answer	Frame
fixation (of)	41. Oophor/o/pexy means fixation of a displaced ovary. -*Pexy* is a suffix meaning ____________.
oophor/o/pexy oophoropexy o͞o′ fôr ō pek′ sē	42. When an ovary is displaced, a surgical procedure to fix it back in its normal place is called ________ / ____ / ______.
oophoropexy	43. The surgical procedure to correct the position of a prolapsed (dropped or sagging) ovary is called an ____________.
fallopian tube(s)	44. *Salping/o* is used to build terms that refer to the fallopian tube(s). A salpingoscope is an instrument used to examine the ________________.
	45. Using what you need of salping/o, build a word meaning
salping/itis salpingitis sal pin jī′ tis	inflammation of a fallopian tube ________ / ______
salping/ectomy salpingectomy sal pin jek′ tō mē	excision of a fallopian tube __________ / __________
salping/ostomy salpingostomy sal pin gos′ tō mē	a permanent opening into a fallopian tube __________ / __________
game and good (pronounce them)	46. In words built from laryng/o, pharyng/o, and salping/o, the "g" is pronounced as a hard "g" *when followed by an "o" or an "a."* The "g" in good is a hard "g." For example, in laryngalgia and salpingocele, the "g" of the word root is pronounced hard as in ________ ________________________. (game/good) or (germ/giant)
hard (pronounce them)	47. In laryngostomy, pharyngotomy, and salpingopexy, the "g" is followed by an "o" and is a __________________ ________________ sound. (hard/soft)
"o" and "a"	48. A hard "g" precedes the vowels ______ and ______.

49.
In words built from laryng/o, pharyng/o, and salping/o, the "g" is soft *when followed by an "e" or an "i"*; for example, in laryngectomy and salpingitis, the "g" is soft as in ____.
(game/good) or (germ/giant)

germ and giant (pronounce them)

50.
In salpingian, laryngitis, and pharyngectomy, the "g" is given a ________________________ sound because it
(soft/hard)
precedes the vowels ________ and ________.

soft (pronounce them)
"e" and "i"

51.
Pronounce each of the following terms.

laryngectomy	pharyngitis
pharyngalgia	salpingo-oophorectomy

In each of the above terms circle the vowel that makes the "g" soft.

laryngectomy
lar in jek′ tō mē
pharyngalgia
far ing gal′ jē a
pharyngitis
far in jī′ tis
salpingo-oophorectomy
sal pin′ gō o͞o fôr ek′ tō mē

52.
In compound medical words, if two like vowels occur between word roots, they are separated by a hyphen. Use salpingo-oophorectomy as a model and build a word that means inflammation of the fallopian tube and ovary:
____________ / ________ / ____________ / ________.

salping/o-/oophor/ itis
salpingo-oophoritis
sal′ pin gō o͞o fôr ī′ tis

53.
Explain when a hyphen (-) is used in compound terms.
____
____
____

Use a hyphen between two like vowels when joining word roots.

54.
Colp/o is used in words about the vagina. Colpitis means ________
____.

inflammation of the vagina

Answer	Frame
	55.
vaginal spasm	A colp/o/spasm is a ____________.
colp/otomy colpotomy kôl pot′ ō mē	Incision into the vagina is a ________ / ________.
	56. Build a word meaning
colp/o/plasty (you pronounce)	surgical repair of the vagina ________ / ____ / ____________
colp/o/scope colposcope kôl′ pō skōp	instrument for examining and visually enlarging vagina ________ / ____ / ____________
	57.
uterus	Hyster/o is used to build words about the uterus. A hyster/ectomy is an excision, or surgical removal, of the ____________.
	58. Write words for the following:
hysterotomy	an incision into the uterus ____________
hysterospasm	a spasm of the uterus ____________
hysteropexy	surgical fixation of the uterus ____________
	59. See Figure 4.2, The Female Reproductive Organs. Examination of the female genital system begins at the vulva (external genitalia), then the vagina, and on to the uterus, fallopian tubes, and ovaries.
hystero/salpingo/ oophor/ectomy	Follow the same order and build a word that means an operation to remove the uterus, fallopian tubes, and ovaries: ________________________________.
	60. Stop here and summarize what you've just covered. Match the best definition in List B with the word root in List A. Write your selection in the space provided.

	LIST A	LIST B
ovary	oophor/o ________________	fallopian tubes
male germ cells	spermat/o ________________	vagina
uterus	hyster/o ________________	male germ cells
fallopian tubes	salping/o ________________	egg, ovum
testicle	orchid/o ________________	hidden
vagina	colp/o ________________	testicle
egg, ovum	o/o ________________	ovary
hidden	crypt ________________	uterus
surgical fixation	-pexy ________________	resembling
produce, originate	-genesis ________________	twitching, spasm
resembling	-oid ________________	suturing to repair
twitching, spasm	-spasm ________________	produce, originate
germ cell, immature cell	-blast ________________	germ cell, immature cell
suturing to repair	-orrhaphy ________________	surgical fixation

61.

Build a word for each of the following:

colp/orrhaphy

suturing (to repair) the vagina ____________ / ________________

hystero/spasm

spasm of the uterus ________________ / ______________

orchido/pexy

fixation of the testis ________________ / ____________

salpingo/oophor/itis

inflammation of ovary and fallopian tube
________________ / ______________ / ____________

spermato/genesis

formation of spermatozoa
____________________ / ________________

spermato/blast

(immature) male germ cell
____________________ / ______________

62.

Now let's have some fun. Read each term and its meaning. Then study the accompanying illustrations.

Hernia is the protrusion of an organ, or part of an organ, through the wall of the cavity that normally contains it; a rupture.

Ptosis is the sinking down or sagging of an organ or part (from its normal position).

Anomaly is an irregularity. It is an organ or structure that is abnormal or contrary to the general rule.

Aneurysm is a localized abnormal dilation of a blood vessel, or ballooning out of the vessel at a weak point.

Write the correct term below each illustration:

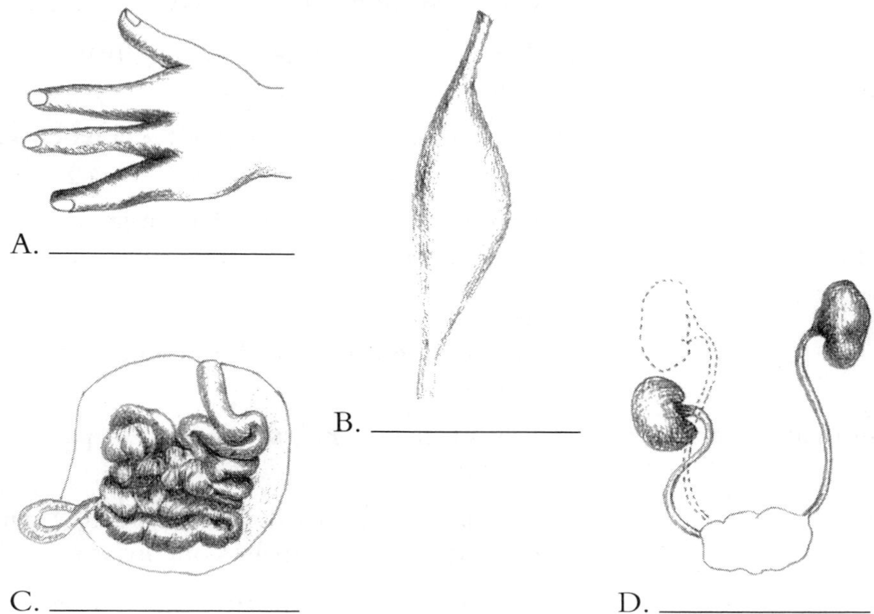

A. anomaly
B. aneurysm
C. hernia
D. ptosis

Figure 4.3

63.

Hyster/o/ptosis means prolapse (sagging) or sinking down of the uterus. Ptosis (pronounced tō′ sis) is a word that means ______________ ______________.

sinking down, prolapse, or sagging

64.

Upon examination, a physician may find that a patient's uterus has prolapsed or moved lower in the pelvic region. The medical term describing this condition is ______________ / ______ / ______________.

hyster/o/ptosis

When uterine prolapse occurs, a surgeon may surgically replace the uterus to its normal position. A hysteropexy would be done to correct or repair the condition known as ______________ / ______ / ______________.

hyster/o/ptosis
hysteroptosis
his′ ter op tō′ sis

65.
From the terms provided, select one that best fits each definition.

anomaly hernia aneurysm ptosis

Protrusion of an organ or part through the wall of the cavity in which it is normally enclosed. ______________

hernia

The prolapse, or sagging, of an organ or part from its normal position. ______________

ptosis

The abnormal ballooning out of a blood vessel at a weak point. ______________

aneurysm

Irregularity in structure of an organ or part; the structure is contrary to the general rule. ______________

anomaly

66.
Fill in the missing words to complete each of the following definitions.

Ptosis is the sagging of an organ or part from its ______________ position.

normal

Hernia is the protrusion of an organ or part through the ________ of a cavity that normally contains it.

wall

Anomaly is an irregularity. It is an organ or structure that is contrary to the ____________.

rule

Aneurysm is the abnormal ballooning out at a weak point in a ______________ ______________.

blood vessel

67.
Complete each of the following descriptions by writing the form of the term that fits best.

An irregular organ or structure that is contrary to the general rule is said to be ______________.

anomalous (adjective)
an anomaly (noun)

When an organ or part protrudes through the wall of the cavity that normally contains it, we say it has ______________.

herniated (verb)

When a weak spot in the wall of the aorta (artery) balloons out, we call it an aortic ______________.

aneurysm (noun)

Nephr/o is used in words that refer to the kidney. If a kidney sags from its normal position, the medical condition is referred to as ____________ / _____ / ____________.

nephr/o/ptosis

Write the correct term below each illustration:

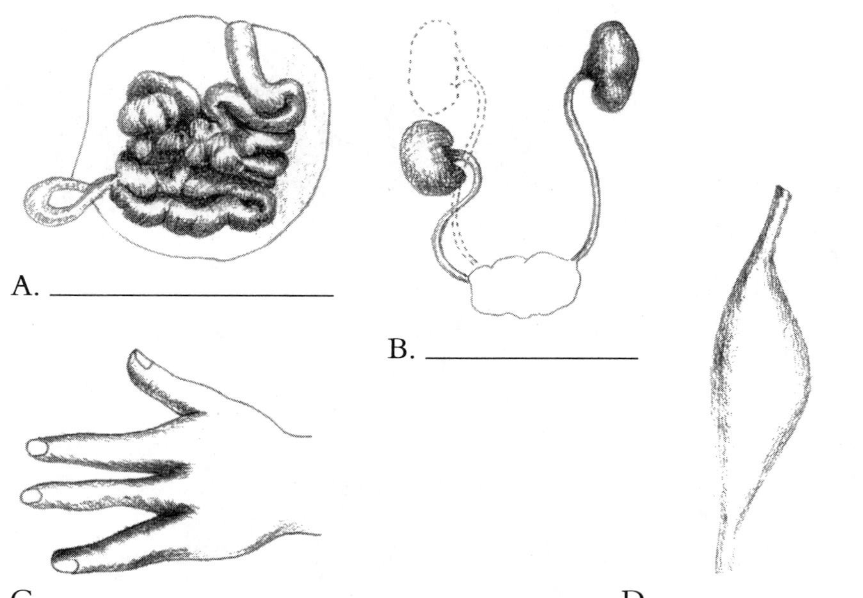

A. ____________

B. ____________

C. ____________

D. ____________

Figure 4.4

A. hernia
B. ptosis
C. anomaly
D. aneurysm

68.
In your own words, write a brief definition for each of the following terms.

aneurysm: ____
____.

anomaly: ____
____.

hernia: ____
____.

ptosis: ____
____.

We suggest something like these:

aneurysm: an abnormal ballooning out of a blood vessel at a weak point.

anomaly: an organ or structure that is contrary to the rule.

hernia: protrusion of an organ or part through the wall that normally contains it.

ptosis: sagging of an organ or part from its normal location.

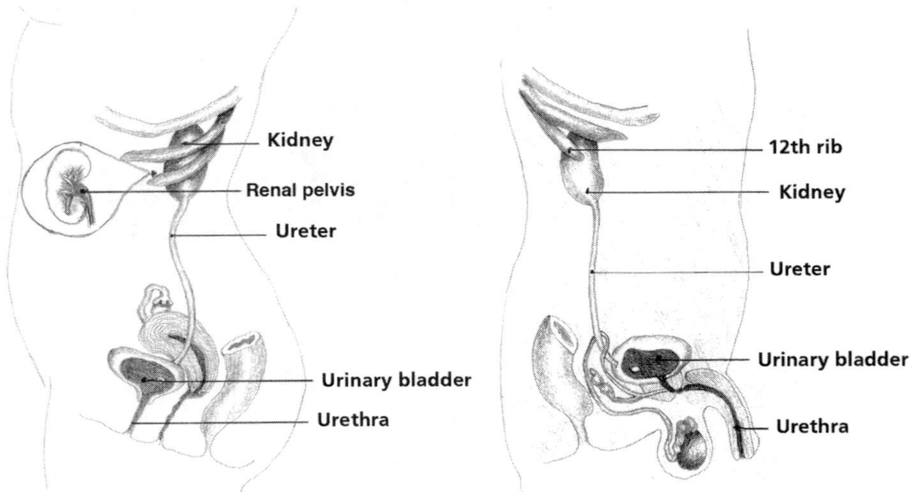

Figure 4.5 The Female Urinary Tract **Figure 4.6** The Male Urinary Tract

The urinary system involves elimination of waste, toxic products, and surplus materials from the body. It also regulates the water and salt content of the body. The urinary tract consists of paired *kidneys* and *ureters,* a single *urinary bladder,* and a urethra. The main organs of excretion are the kidneys. The kidneys are bean-shaped organs about the size of a fist. They are located on either side of the spinal column and usually extend from the 12th rib. One kidney touches the spleen and the other is slightly below the liver. A ureter exits each kidney at the *renal pelvis.* This tube carries urine to the main storage organ, the urinary bladder. The bladder is a hollow muscular sac located in the midline at the floor of the pelvic cavity. It can hold as much as 700-1000 ml of urine without injury. As it distends, it rises into the abdominal cavity. The tube leading from the bladder to the exterior is the *urethra.* This tube is about one and a half inches long in the female and about eight inches long in the male as it passes through the penis.

kidney (nephr/o)	renal pelvis (pyle/o)
bladder (cyst/o)	ureter (ureter/o)
urethra (urethr/o)	urine (ur/o)

69.
Let's go on to a new but related area of the body. Here is a brief summary of the functions of each part of the urinary tract.

kidney:	forms urine
renal pelvis:	collects urine in the kidney
ureter:	carries urine to the bladder
bladder:	stores urine until voiding
urethra:	discharges urine from the body

ur
ur/o

70.
The urinary system is responsible for making urine from waste materials in the blood and carrying urine from the body. What is the word root for urine? ________ What is the combining form? ________

renal pelvis

71.
Pyel/o is the combining form that refers to the ____________________.

pyel/itis
pyelitis
pī ə lī′ tis

pyel/o/plasty
pyeloplasty
pī′ e lō plas tē

72.
Taking what you need from the combining form for renal pelvis, form a term meaning

inflammation of the renal pelvis
____________ / ____________

surgical repair of the renal pelvis
____________ / _____ / ________________

abnormal condition of the renal pelvis and kidney

pyel/o/nephr/itis
pyelonephritis
pī′ lō nef rī′ tis

73.
Pyel/o/nephr/osis means ____
____
____.

Form a term that means inflammation of the renal pelvis and kidney:
____________ / _____ / ________________ / ____________.

stone or calculus in the ureter

74.
Look at Figures 4.5 and 4.6. Ureter/o/lith means ______________
____.

ureter/o/lith/otomy ureterolithotomy	Form a term that means incision into the ureter (for removal of a stone): ________ (ureter) / ____ / ________ (calculus) / ________ (incision into).
surgical repair of the ureter and renal pelvis	75. Ureter/o/pyel/o/plasty means ________________________________.
ureter/o/pyel/itis ureteropyelitis yo͞o rē′ ter ō pī ə lī′ tis	76. Form a term meaning inflammation of the ureter and renal pelvis: ________ / ____ / ________ / ________.
ureter/o/cyst/ostomy ureterocystostomy yo͞o rē′ ter ō sis tos′ tō mē	77. Form a term that means making a permanent opening between the ureter and bladder: ________ (ureter) / ____ / ________ (bladder) / ________ (permanent opening).
	78. *Orrhaphy* is not really a suffix, but again (for simplification) it can be used as one. Orrhaphy means suturing or stitching (for the purpose of repair, especially after trauma). Form a word meaning
ureter/orrhaphy ureterorrhaphy yer rē ter ôr′ ə fē	suturing of the ureter ________ / ________
nephr/orrhaphy nephrorrhaphy nef rôr′ ə fē	suturing of a kidney ________ / ________
cyst/orrhaphy cystorrhaphy sis tôr′ ə fē	suturing the bladder ________ / ________
neur/orrhaphy neurorrhaphy nyo͞o rôr′ ə fē	suturing of a nerve ________ / ________

Answers	Frames
	79.
to carry urine out of the body or remove urine from the bladder	Look back at Figures 4.5 and 4.6. What is the function of the urethra? ______________________ ______________________ ______________________
urethr-	What is the word root for urethra? ______________
suturing of the urethra (to repair)	Urethr/orrhaphy means ______________________ ______________.
	80. Form a word that means
urethr/otomy urethrotomy yer ə throt′ ə mē	incision into the urethra ________ / ________
urethr/o/spasm urethrospasm yer rē′ thrō spasm	spasm of the urethra ________ / ____ / ________
	81. Another complex word part is -orrhagia, which can be used as a suffix when it follows a word root. *Orrhagia* means bursting forth of blood (as in hemorrhage).
	Build a word that means
cyst/orrhagia cystorrhagia sis tō rä′ jē ə	bursting forth of blood from the bladder ________ / ________
ureter/orrhagia ureterorrhagia yer rē′ ter ō rä′ jē ə	hemorrhage of the ureter ________ / ________ (ureter / bursting forth of blood)
	82. Di/a is the combining form meaning pass through or secrete freely.
	Define: (Use your dictionary.)
	diuresis ______________________
(How does the dictionary define these terms?)	diuretic ______________________
	dialysis ______________________

83.

Let's have a brief review. Select the correct word root or suffix from List B. Write your selection in the space provided in List A.

	LIST A	LIST B
cyst/o-	stores urine until voiding ________	nephr/o-
aneurysm	ballooning-out vessel ________	pyel/o-
ureter/o-	carries urine to bladder ________	urethr/o-
anomaly	contrary to the rule, irregular ________	ur/o-
pyel/o-	collects urine in the kidney ________	ureter/o-
urethr/o-	discharges urine from body ________	cyst/o-
neur/o-	nerve ________	aneurysm
hernia	protrusion through cavity wall ________	anomaly
ur/o-	urine ________	hernia
nephr/o-	forms urine ________	neur/o-
-plasty	surgical repair (make new) ________	-lith
-ptosis	drooping, prolapse ________	-plasty
-pexy	fixing in place ________	-ptosis
-lith	stone, calculus ________	-orrhaphy
-orrhaphy	suturing to repair ________	-orrhagia
-ostomy	permanent opening ________	-ostomy
-orrhagia	hemorrhage ________	-spasm
-spasm	twitching, muscle cramp ________	-pexy

84.

Build a word for each of the following definitions.

pyelo/nephr/osis

diseased condition of renal pelvis and kidney
________ / ________ / ________

uretero/lith/otomy

incision to remove calculus from ureter
________ / ________ / ________

nephro/ptosis

sagging of the kidney
________ / ________

ur/ology

the study of urine and the urinary system
________ / ________

ureter/orrhaphy

suturing, reconnection of the ureter
________ / ________

nephro/plasty

repair (make new) the kidney
________ / ________

cyst/orrhagia

hemorrhage from the urinary bladder
________ / ________

nephro/pexy

surgical fixing of the kidney in its place
________ / ________

85.

Following are 46 of the medical terms you formed in Chapter 4. Pronounce each one aloud and spell it on paper.

aneurysm (an′yo͞o rizm)
angioblast (an′ jē ō blast)
angiosclerosis
  (an′ jē ō sklə rō′ sis)
anomaly (an om′ə lē)
apnea (ap′ nē ə)
arteriosclerosis
  (ar ter′ ē ō skler ō′ sis)
arteriospasm
  (ar ter′ ē ō spa′zm)
colporrhaphy (kôl pōr′ə fē)
colposcopy (kôl pōs′ kō pē)
cryptorchidism
  (krip′ ôr kid ism)
cystorrhagia (sis tō rä jē ə)
dysmenorrhea
  (dis′ men ōr rē′ ə)
dyspepsia (dis pep′sē ə)
dyspnea (disp′ nē ə)
hemangiitis (hē man jē ī′tis)
hematologist (hē mə tol′ ō jist)
hemolysis (hē mol′ ə sis)
hernia (her′ nē ə)
hysteropexy (his′ter ō peks′ ē)
hysterospasm (his′ter ō spa zm)
hysterotomy (his ter ot′ ō mē)
kinesialgia (kin ē′ sē al′ jē ə)
kinesiology (kin ē′ sē ol′ ə jē)

myosclerosis (mī ō skler ō′ sis)
myospasm (mī′ ō spa zm)
nephritis (nef rī′tis)
nephrolith (nef′rō lith)
nephromegaly (nef′rō meg ə lē)
nephroptosis (nef rop tō′ sis)
neurofibroma
  (nyo͞o′ rō fī brō′ mä)
neurolysis (nyo͞o rol′ ə sis)
o-oblast (ō′ō blast)
oophoropexy (o͞o′ fôr ō pek′ sē)
orchidotomy (or kid ot′ ō mē)
pyelitis (pī ə lī′ tis)
pyeloplasty (pī′ ə lō plas tē)
salpingectomy
  (sal pin jek′ tō mē)
salpingo-oophorectomy
  (sal pin′ gō o͞o fôr ek′ tō mē)
salpingoscopy (sal pin gos′ kō pē)
spermatoblast (sper mat′ ō blast)
spermatoid (sper′ ma toid)
ureterolithotomy
  (yer rē′ ter ō lith ot′ ō mē)
ureterorrhaphy
  (yer rē ter ôr′ ə fē)
ureterotomy (yer ē ter ot′ə mē)
urethralgia (yer ə thral′ jē ə)
urethrotomy (yer e throt′ ə mē)

Complete the Chapter 4 Self-Test before going to the next unit.

Chapter 4 Self-Test

Part 1

From the list on the right, select the correct meaning for each of the following terms:

______ 1. Urethrospasm
______ 2. Spermatoid
______ 3. Nephroptosis
______ 4. Anomaly
______ 5. Oophoropexy
______ 6. Angioblast
______ 7. Ureterotomy
______ 8. Angiosclerosis
______ 9. Hysterotomy
______ 10. Myospasm
______ 11. Dyspepsia
______ 12. Hemolysis
______ 13. Kinesiology
______ 14. Aneurysm

a. The study (or science) of motion
b. A condition of hardening of vessels
c. Spasm of the urethra
d. Destruction of blood (cells)
e. Surgical fixation of the ovary in its place
f. Tumor of nerve and fibrous tissue
g. Muscle spasm
h. Structure contrary to the rule
i. Resembling sperm
j. Abnormally enlarged kidney
k. Ballooning out of blood vessel
l. Painful menstruation (cramps)
m. Vessel germ cell
n. Kidney out of its normal place (dropped kidney)
o. Incision into the uterus (cesarean section)
p. Painful digestion (heartburn)
q. Incision into the ureter

Part 2

Complete each of the medical terms on the right with the appropriate missing part:

1. A condition of hardening of muscle ________ sclerosis
2. Kidney stone Nephro ________
3. Painful menstruation ________ menorrhea
4. Spasm of the uterus ________ spasm
5. Cessation of menses A ________
6. Hemorrhage (bleeding) from the bladder ________ orrhagia
7. Surgical removal of the ovary ________ ectomy
8. Incision into the ureter (for the purpose of removing a stone) ________ lithotomy
9. Surgical removal of the fallopian tube ________ ectomy
10. Drooping of an organ P ________
11. Pain due to motion ________ algia
12. Spasm of the vessels ________ spasm
13. Protrusion of an organ through a cavity wall H ________
14. Incision into the urethra ________ otomy

ANSWERS

Part 1	*Part 2*
1. c	1. Myosclerosis
2. j	2. Nephrolith
3. o	3. Dysmenorrhea
4. i	4. Hysterospasm
5. f	5. Amenorrhea
6. n	6. Cystorrhagia
7. r	7. Oophorectomy
8. b	8. Ureterolithotomy

9. p	9. Salpingectomy
10. h	10. Ptosis
11. q	11. Kinesialgia
12. d	12. Angiospasm
13. a	13. Hernia
14. l	14. Urethrotomy

5 The Gastrointestinal Tract

In Chapter 5 you'll make more than 50 new medical terms. Most of the learning material focuses on terms relating to the gastrointestinal (GI) tract. Three illustrations provide information you'll need as you work through the learning sequences and exercises. Be sure to bookmark those illustrations and keep them handy. Use them often.

Chapter 5 addresses the gastrointestinal system. Broken down, "gastrointestinal" indicates the gastric area, or the stomach, and the intestinal area immediately following the stomach to the anus, the outlet of the GI system or tract. This section of the head-to-toe assessment provides information about the health of these organs and the function of digestion and bowel elimination, including potential problems. Closely tied to the GI assessment is the abdominal assessment. These two areas are anatomically so close together that they may even be documented in one section of a head-to-toe assessment, providing data about masses, tenderness, and abnormalities inside the abdomen. This section will also include information about the liver, gall bladder, pancreas, spleen, and vascular sounds (sounds arising from blood flow) in the abdomen and kidneys. Let's get started learning terms associated with these areas.

Mini-Glossary

Root Words

cheil/o (*lip, lips*)
col/o (*colon*)
dent/o (*teeth*)
esophag/o (*esophagus*)
gingiv/o (*gums*)
gloss/o (*tongue*)
hepat/o (*liver*)
pancreat/o (*pancreas*)
proct/o (*anus and rectum*)
rect/o (*rectum*)
stomat/o (*mouth*)

Suffixes

-clysis (*irrigation*)
-ectasia (*dilation, stretching*)
-scope, -scopy (*look, examine*)
-toxin (*poison*)

Take a few minutes to complete the Review Sheet for Chapter 4 before you begin Chapter 5.

1.
You're going to begin this section with a review of suffixes you have already studied and used.

Write the meaning of each of the following:

of, or pertaining to	-ic, -as, -ar ________
surgical repair, make new, restore	-plasty ________
inflammation of	-itis ________
twitching, cramping	-spasm ________
pain, ache	-algia ________
under, beneath	-hypo ________
excessive, too much	-hyper ________
surgical excision of	-ectomy ________
incision into	-otomy ________
bursting forth, hemorrhage	-orrhagia ________
a noun ending meaning condition, condition of	-a, -ia ________
abnormal condition, diseased condition	-osis ________

2.
This time, write the suffix that satisfies each of the definitions given. Then go back to the last frame to check your answers.

MEANING	SUFFIX
pain, ache	________
excessive, too much	________
surgical incision into	________
inflammation of	________
under, beneath	________
twitching, cramping	________
surgical excision of	________
bursting forth, hemorrhage	________
of, or pertaining to	________
an ending meaning condition	________
abnormal (diseased) condition	________

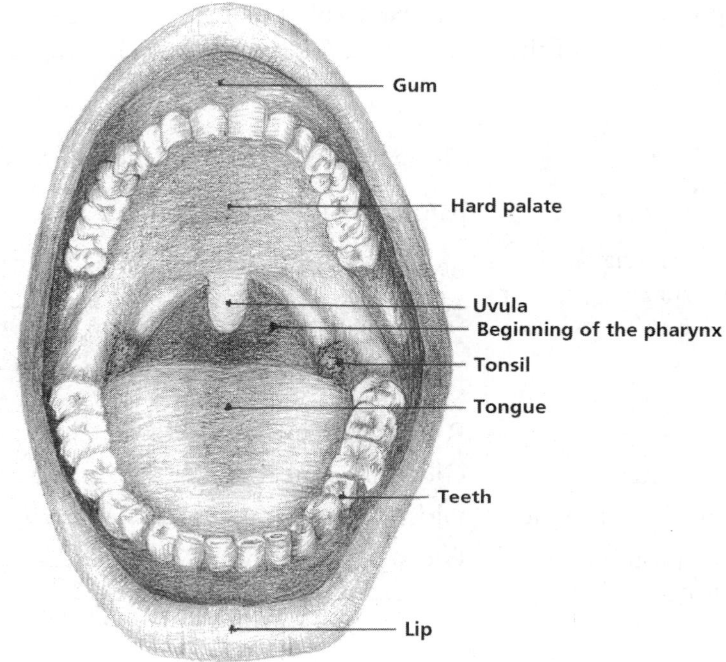

Figure 5.1 The Oral Cavity

The digestive tract begins at the mouth, the oral cavity. The human mouth is concerned with vocalization as well as mastication (chewing) and swallowing. The anterior portion includes lips, teeth, gums, a muscular tongue, related muscles, salivary glands, a bony palate, and muscles of the cheek wall. All are concerned with wetting, macerating, and pulverizing ingested material. The posterior portion of the oral cavity includes the soft palate, tongue, tonsils, and taste buds.

mouth (stomat/o)
tongue (gloss/o)
lip (cheil/o)
gum (gingiv/o)
tooth (dent/o)

stomat
stomat/o

3.
The word root for mouth is ____________________.
The combining form is ____________________ / ________.

inflammation of the mouth

4.
Stomat/itis means ____.

surgical repair or reconstruction of the mouth	Stomat/o/plast/y means ______________________________ ______________________________.
	5.
stomat/algia stomatalgia stō mä tal′ jē ə	Using the word root for mouth, form a word meaning painful mouth ______________ / ______________
stomat/orrhagia stomatorrhagia stō mat′ ō rä′ jē ə	hemorrhage of the mouth ______________ / ______________ mouth hemorrhage
	6. Refer to Figure 5.1.
painful tongue	Gloss/algia means ______________________________.
excision of the tongue	Gloss/ectomy means ______________________________.
spasm or twitching of the tongue	Gloss/o/spasm means ______________________________ ______________________________.
	7.
gloss/itis glossitis glos ī′ tis	Using the word root, build a term meaning inflammation of the tongue ______________ / ______________
gloss/al glossal glos′ əl	pertaining to the tongue ______________ / __________
	8.
hypo/gloss/al hypoglossal hī′ pō glos′ əl	What word would you use to describe a medication that is administered under the tongue? ______________ / ______________ / __________ under tongue pertaining to
	9.
cheil cheil/o kē′ lō	Go back to Figure 5.1. The word root for lip is ______________. The combining form for lip is ______________ / _______.
	10.
inflammation of the lips	Cheil/itis means ______________________________ ______________________________.
plastic surgery of the lips	Cheil/o/plast/y means ______________________________ ______________________________.

cheil/otomy
cheilotomy
kē lot′ ō mē

cheil/osis
cheilosis
kē lō′ sis

11.
Build a term meaning

incision into the lips _______________ / _______________

abnormal condition or diseased condition of the lips
_______________ / _______________

cheil/o/stomat/o/plasty
cheilostomatoplasty
kē′ lō stō mat′ ō plas tē

12.
Now, build a term meaning plastic surgery of the lips and mouth:
__________ / _____ / _______________ / _____ /__________.
lip mouth repair

gingiv/o
of or pertaining to gums

13.
The combining form for gums is _______________ / _____.
Gingival means _______________________________________.

gingiv/itis
gingivitis
jin ji vī′ tis

gingiv/algia
gingivalgia
jin ji val′ jē ə

gingiv/ectomy
gingivectomy
jin ji vek′ tə mē

gingiv/o/gloss/itis
gingivoglossitis
jin′ ji vō glos ī′ tis

14.
Build a term meaning

inflammation of the gums _______________ / _______________

painful gums _______________ / _______________

excision of gum tissue _______________ / _______________

inflammation of the gums and tongue
_______________ / _____ / _______________ / __________

inflammation of the gums
surgical excision of the tongue
toothache
plastic surgery, repair of the lips
hemorrhage of the mouth

15.
Here's a quick review. Without referring to the tables, write a meaning for each of the following.

gingivitis _______________________________________

glossectomy _______________________________________

dentalgia _______________________________________

cheiloplasty _______________________________________

stomatorrhagia _______________________________________

16.
Using the suggested word roots, make a medical term that fits each definition below.

SUGGESTED ANSWERS:
stomat-
cheil-
gingiv-
gloss-
dent-

Answer	Definition
glossitis	inflammation of the tongue ________
cheilosis	abnormal, diseased condition of the lips ________
dentalgia	toothache ________
stomatoplasty	plastic surgery, repair of the mouth ________
gingivectomy	surgical excision of gum tissue ________

Take a break. You deserve it.

17.
Again, you will use many suffixes you are already familiar with. Here's an opportunity to refresh your memory. See how many you can correctly define. Write your answers in the space provided.

Answer	Suffix
puncture of cavity, to withdraw fluid	-centesis ________
incision into	-otomy ________
form a new (permanent) opening	-ostomy ________
study of	-ology ________
surgical fixation of a part in its normal place	-pexy ________
hernia, herniation	-cele ________
calculus, stone	-lith ________
large, enlarged	-megaly ________

18.

Now, complete the table below. You will use it in the next few frames. Write the suffix that satisfies the definition given. Check your answers in frame 17.

Meaning	**Suffix**
calculus, stone	-________________
surgical fixation of a part in place	-________________
incision into	-________________
study of	-________________
hernia, herniation	-________________
large, enlarged	-________________
form a new opening (permanent)	-________________
puncture a cavity and draw fluid	-________________

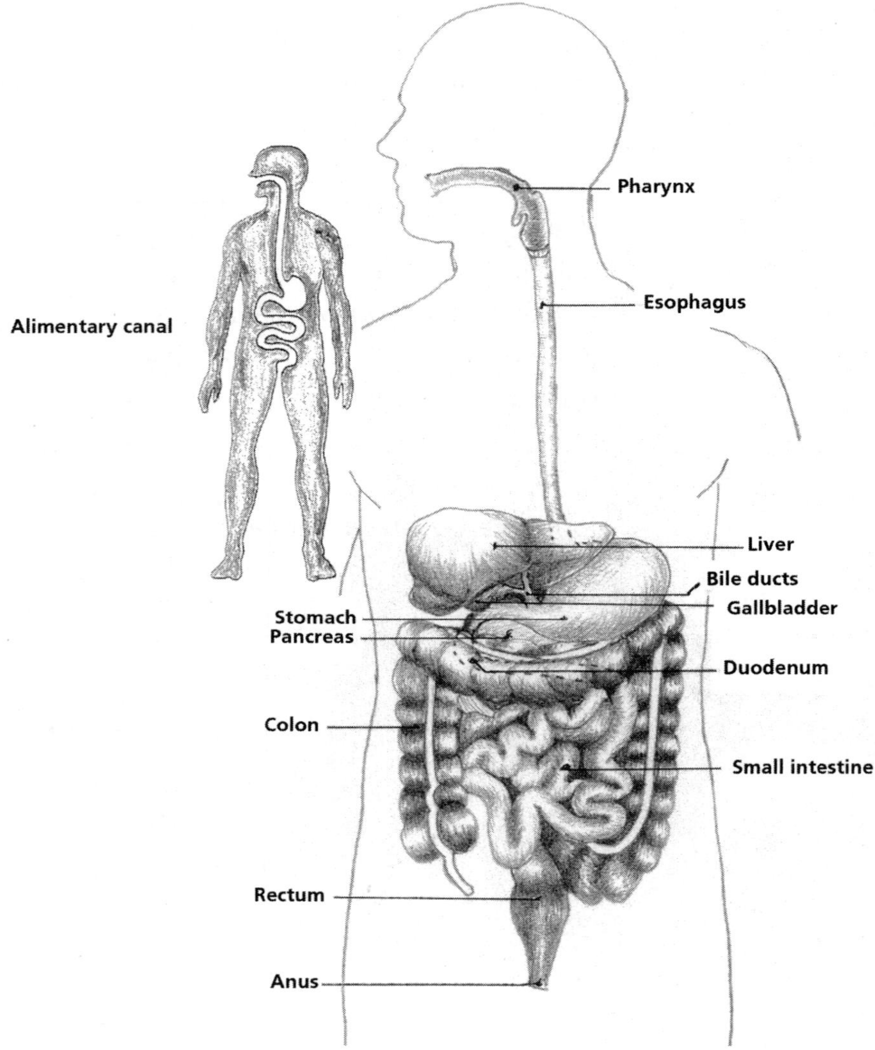

Figure 5.2 The Digestive Tract

The function of the digestive system is to break down large food particles into smaller ones that can pass across the membranes of cells and be absorbed. The digestive tract, also known as the *alimentary canal*, consists of a single long tube extending from mouth to anus and opened to the exterior at each end. The canal begins with the oral cavity. Here the teeth pulverize ingested food. Meanwhile it is softened and partly digested by salivary gland secretions. The tongue aids in mechanical manipulation of the food and literally flips the food into the fibromuscular *pharynx* during swallowing. The *esophagus* moves the food bolus along to the pouchlike *stomach* by peristaltic muscular contractions. Here the food mixes with acid and protein-digesting enzymes and is retained until digested further. Passing from the stomach, the food enters the first part of the small intestine, called the *duodenum*. Liver-produced bile, stored in the *gallbladder,* is discharged into the duodenum by *bile ducts*. Digestive enzymes from the *pancreas* enter the duodenum as well. The food bolus continues through the highly coiled 20-foot-long *small intestine*. A great portion of the abdominal cavity is taken up by the many folds and twists of this organ. Small molecular nutrients are extracted and absorbed by cells lining the intestine. These nutrients absorbed throughout the tract are transferred to capillaries and transported to the *liver* by the hepatic portal system for processing and distribution to the body's cells. The *colon* or large intestine can be seen ascending along the anatomical right side, passing across the midline, then turning and descending along the left. This organ is mainly concerned with absorption of water, minerals, and certain vitamins. The non-nutritive residue of the ingested food is compacted and moved through the *rectum* and the *anal canal* to the outside.

liver (hepat/o)
pharynx (pharyng/o)
esophagus (esophag/o)
intestine (enter/o)
rectum and anus (proct/o)
rectum (rect/o)
stomach (gastr/o)
gallbladder (cholecyst/o)
duodenum (duoden/o)
colon (col/o)
pancreas (pancreat/o)
anus (an/o)

19.

Answer	Frame
stomach hemorrhage	Here are some easy ones. Gastr/orrhagia means ________________.
inflammation of the stomach	Gastritis means ________________________________.
of, or pertaining to, the stomach	Gastric means ________________________________.

20.

Here are some new suffixes.

-ectasia means dilation, stretching, or expansion
-clysis means irrigation, or washing out
-toxin means poison, or poisoning

Use Figure 5.2 and write a meaning for the following medical terms.

Answer	Frame
poisoning of the small intestine	enter/o/toxin ________________________________
stretching, dilation of the small intestine	enter/ectasia ________________________________
irrigation, washing out of the small intestine	enter/o/clysis ________________________________

21.

Answer	Frame
washing, irrigation of the colon	What do you think col/o/clysis means? ________________________________
dilation, stretching, or expanding of the stomach	What does gastr/ectasia mean? ________________________________

22.

Use Figure 5.2 as you need to, and try these.

Answer	Frame
a surgical procedure to fix the colon in its normal place	col/o/pexy means ________________________________.
herniation of the small intestine	enter/o/cele means ________________________________.
a surgical procedure to make a new (permanent) opening into the colon	col/ostomy means ________________________________.

	23.
gastr/o/enter/ostomy gastroenterostomy gas′ trō en ter os′ tō mē	Form a term describing a surgical procedure that forms a new opening between the stomach and small intestine _______ / ___ / _______ / _______
gastr/o/enter/ic gastroenteric gas′ trō en ter′ ik	pertaining to the stomach and small intestine _______ / ___ / _______ / _____
	24.
enter/o/clysis enteroclysis en ter ok′ li sis	Refer to Figure 5.2 again. Build a term meaning washing or irrigation of the small intestine _______ / ___ / _______
enter/ectasia enterectasia en′ ter ek tā′ jē ə	dilation of the small intestine _______ / _______
	25.
	What do the following terms mean?
poisoning of the small intestine	enter/o/toxin ______________
puncture of the small intestine, to withdraw fluid	enter/o/centesis ______________
intestinal hernia	enter/o/cele ______________
	26.
	Try these.
pertaining to the colon or large intestine	col/ic ______________
puncture of the colon, draw fluid	col/o/centesis ______________
making a permanent opening into the colon	col/ostomy ______________
	27.
col/o/pexy colopexy kō′ lō pek sē	Build a term meaning surgical fixation of the colon _______ / ___ / _______

col/o/clysis
coloclysis
kō lok′ li sis

washing or irrigation of the colon
__________ / _____ / ______________

col/itis
colitis
kō lī′ tis

inflammation of the colon __________ / ____________

28.
Refer to Figure 5.2 again. The combining form for rectum is ____________ / _____.

rect/o

What does each of the following mean?

pertaining to the rectum

rect/al ____

a rectal hernia

rect/o/cele ____

washing or irrigation of the rectum (enema)

rect/o/clysis ____

29.
Build a word meaning

rect/o/colitis
rectocolitis
rek′ tō kō li′ tis

inflammation of the rectum and colon
____________ / _____ / __________________

rect/o/cyst/otomy
rectocystotomy
rek′ tō sis tot′ ə mē

incision of the bladder through the rectum
____________ / _____ / ____________ / ________________
rectum / bladder / incision into

30.
Proctology is the study of diseases of the anus and rectum. A proct/o/log/ist is one who ____.

specializes in diseases of the anus and rectum

31.
Build a word meaning washing or irrigation of anus and rectum:
________________ / _____ / ________________.

proct/o/clysis
proctoclysis (enema)

prok tok′ li sis

Pronounce that one several times.

32.
Write a meaning for each of the following:

instrument for examining the anus and rectum
prok′ tə skōp

proct/o/scope ____

examination of the anus and rectum prok tos′ kō pē	proct/o/scopy ______________________________ ______________________________
	33. Back to Figure 5.2. What is the combining form for liver?
hepat/o	______________
pertaining to the liver	Hepat/ic means ______________________________.
an abnormal condition of enlargement of the liver	Hepatomegaly means ______________________________ ______________________________.
	34. Build a word meaning
hepat/o/scop/y hepatoscopy hep ə tos′ kō pē	inspection (examination) of the liver __________ / ____ / __________ / ____
hepat/otomy hepatotomy hep ə tot′ ō mē	incision into the liver __________ / __________
hepat/itis hepatitis hep ə tī′ tis	inflammation of the liver __________ / __________
	35.
pertaining to the pancreas	Here's another new term. Pancreat/ic means ______________ ______________________________.
	Underline the part of the term that means dissolution or destruction.
pancreat/o/<u>lysis</u>	pancreat/o/lys/is
	36. Build a word meaning
pancreat/o/lith pancreatolith pan krē at′ ə lith	a stone or calculus in the pancreas __________ / ____ / __________ pancreas stone
pancreat/itis pancreatitis pan krē a tī′ tis	inflammation of the pancreas __________ / __________
pancreat/ectomy pancreatectomy pan krē a tek′ tō mē	excision of part or all of the pancreas __________ / __________
pancreat/otomy pancreatotomy pan krē a tot′ ə mē	incision into the pancreas __________ / __________

37.

When an entire gastrectomy is performed, a new connection (opening) is formed between the esophagus and duodenum. This is called an ______________ / _____ / ___________ / ___________.

(Note: Remember to name the anatomical parts in the order in which food passes through them.)

esophag/o/duoden/ostomy
esophagoduodenostomy
ē sof′ ə gō do͞o′ ō den os′ tō mē

38.

As you rewrite each of the following, analyze it (make your own diagonal divisions) and pronounce it to yourself:

gastroenterocolostomy ______________________________

gastr/o/enter/o/col/ostomy

esophagogastrostomy ______________________________

esophag/o/gastr/ostomy

enterocholecystostomy ______________________________

enter/o/chol/e/cyst/ostomy

39.

Try it again:

proctectasia ______________________________

proct/ectasia

duodenocholecystostomy ______________________________

duoden/o/chol/e/cyst/ostomy

esophagogastroscopy ______________________________

esophag/o/gastr/o/scopy

40.

Let's review what you just covered. Using the suggested answers, write the meaning of each of the following terms.

SUGGESTED ANSWERS:

colon	lips	rectum
duodenum	liver	anus and rectum
esophagus	mouth	small intestine
gums	pancreas	tongue
stomach		

rectum	rect/o ______
colon	col/o ______
pancreas	pancreat/o ______
rectum and anus	proct/o ______
lips	cheil/o ______
mouth	stomat/o ______
small intestine	enter/o ______
esophagus	esophag/o ______
gums	gingiv/o ______
tongue	gloss/o ______
liver	hepat/o ______
duodenum	duoden/o ______
stomach	gastr/o ______

41.
Try these.

SUGGESTED ANSWERS:

make a new opening	stretching
poison	irrigation
look, examine	

irrigation	-clysis ______
look, examine	-scope, -scopy ______
make a new opening	-ostomy ______
stretching	-ectasia ______
poison	-toxin ______

42.

Here's what we suggest:	In your own words, write the meaning of each of the following medical terms.
a new opening between the esophagus and duodenum	esophag/o/duoden/ostomy ______ ______
inspection of the anus and rectum (with an instrument)	proct/oscopy ______ ______

plastic surgery of the lips

cheil/o/plasty

____

____

stretching of the esophagus

esophag/o/ectasia

____

____

irrigation of the anus and rectum (and lower colon; enema)

proct/o/clysis

____

____

pain of the stomach and intestine

gastr/o/enter/algia

____

____

incision into the pancreas

pancreat/otomy

____

____

tumor of the mouth

stomat/oma

____

____

spasm of the tongue

gloss/o/spasm

____

____

an endoscopic exam of the esophagus, stomach, and duodenum

43.
Some terms are composed of many word roots plus a prefix and a suffix. These terms usually list the parts of the body in a special order.

Take a look at Figure 5.3 below. For example, when you swallow food it passes from the mouth to the esophagus to the stomach to the duodenum. So when a physician takes a look inside the digestive system with an endoscope the procedure is called

esophago / gastro / duoden / oscopy

Describe what the procedure EGD means. ______________________________

____

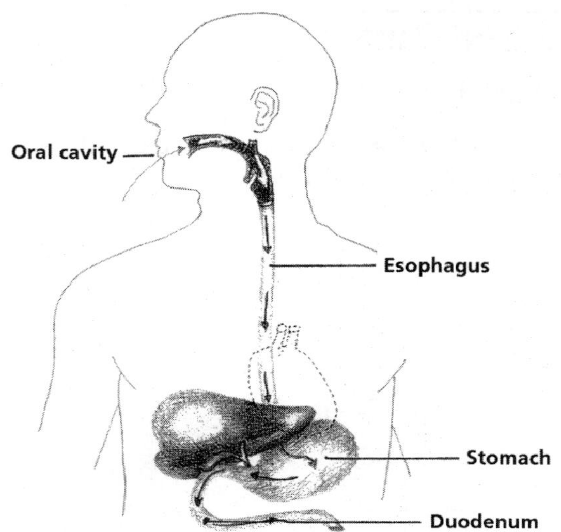

Figure 5.3 Path of EGD Examination

44.
Here are 25 medical terms for practicing your pronunciation. Say the term aloud and then say what it means. Then take the Chapter 5 Self-Test.

cheilitis (kē lī′ tis)
cheiloplasty (kē′ lō plas tē)
colic (kol′ ik)
colitis (kō lī′ tis)
colostomy (kō los′ tō mē)
dentalgia (den tal′ jē ə)
enterocele (en′ ter ō sēl)
enteroclysis (en ter ok′ li sis)
enterotoxin (en′ ter ō tox in)
esophagogastroscopy (ē sof′ ə gō gas tros′ kō pē)
gastrectasia (gas trek tā′ zhə)
gastrorrhagia (gas′ trō rä′ jē ə)
gingivectomy (jin ji vek′ tō mē)
gingivoglossitis (jin′ ji vō glos ī′ tis)
glossospasm (glos′ ō spa zm)
hepatitis (hep a tī′ tis)
hepatomegaly (hep a tō meg′ a lē)
hepatorrhagia (hep a tō rä′ jē a)
hypoglossal (hī′ pō glos′ əl)
pancreatectomy (pan krē a tek′ tō mē)
proctoclysis (prok tok′ li sis)
proctoscopy (prok tos′ kō pē)
rectal (rek′ t'l)
stomatitis (stō mä tī′ tis)
stomatorrhagia (stō mät ō rä′ jē ə)

Chapter 5 Self-Test

Part 1

From the list on the right, select the correct meaning for each of the following often used medical terms.

_____ 1. Proctoclysis
_____ 2. Stomatoplasty
_____ 3. Hepatectomy
_____ 4. Stomatorrhagia
_____ 5. Colic
_____ 6. Enteroclysis
_____ 7. Glossospasm
_____ 8. Dental
_____ 9. Enterotoxin
_____ 10. Cheilitis
_____ 11. Colostomy
_____ 12. Gastrectasia
_____ 13. Cheiloplasty
_____ 14. Hepatomegaly
_____ 15. Proctoscopy

a. Make a new opening in the colon
b. Abnormal enlargement of the liver
c. Of or pertaining to teeth
d. Intestinal poisoning
e. Stretching, dilation of the stomach
f. Spasm of the tongue
g. Hemorrhage of the mouth
h. Irrigation of the rectum and anus
i. Plastic surgery of the mouth
j. Relating to the colon
k. Plastic surgery of the lips
l. Irrigation of the intestine
m. Surgical removal of (part of) the liver
n. Examination (looking into) the rectum through the anus with an endoscope
o. Inflammation of the lips

Part 2

Complete each of the medical terms on the right with the appropriate terms.

1. Under the tongue ________________
2. Surgical removal of the pancreas ________________
3. Hemorrage of the mouth ________________
4. Inflammation of the lips ________________
5. Enlarged liver ________________
6. Stretching or dilation of the stomach ________________
7. Spasm of the tongue ________________
8. Plastic surgery of the lips ________________
9. Intestinal hernia ________________
10. Inflammation of the liver ________________
11. Instrument for examining the rectum and anus ________________
12. Pertaining to the rectum ________________
13. Formation of a new opening in the colon ________________
14. Painful tongue ________________
15. Irrigation of the rectum and anus ________________

ANSWERS

Part 1	*Part 2*
1. h	1. Hypoglossal
2. i	2. Pancreatectomy
3. m	3. Stomatorrhagia
4. g	4. Cheilitis
5. j	5. Hepatomegaly
6. l	6. Gastrectasia
7. f	7. Glossospasm
8. c	8. Cheiloplasty
9. d	9. Enterocele
10. o	10. Hepatitis

11. a	11. Proctoscope
12. e	12. Rectal
13. k	13. Colostomy
14. b	14. Glossalgia
15. n	15. Proctoclysis

6 The Heart

Chapter 6 focuses on the gross anatomy of the heart and how the heart works. You'll create terms relating to abnormal conditions of the heart, and its abnormal functions. You'll also cover some new prefixes and suffixes as shown below.

As you learn the terms associated with the heart, remember that this is another important step in the head-to-toe assessment. As you can imagine, this section includes a lot of important data on a client's health status. The cardiac section includes any problems with the heart, veins, or arteries. Arteries are the vessels that carry blood away from the heart to provide oxygen to the tissues in the body. Veins are the vessels that carry unoxygenated blood back to the heart to pick up more oxygen and discard waste. There will often be an extensive description in the assessment of heart sounds. Abnormal heart sounds are described as murmurs and may be documented. There also may be information on arrhythmias or an abnormal heart rhythm. Depending on the client's history, this section may be brief or extensive.

In this chapter you will also be exposed to many terms involved in the extremity portion of the head-to-toe assessment. The extremities section includes the arms and legs, as the name suggests. Information in this section of the medical record would include peripheral perfusion (or how the blood vessels provide blood to and remove blood from the extremities), capillary refill (whether the smallest of blood vessels are providing and removing blood to the hands and feet), pulses, sensory assessment of the periphery (checking the nerve function for feeling in the arms and legs), mobility assessments (the ability to move), deformations, and any abnormalities in the human periphery. Let's get started learning the new terms associated with this area!

Mini-Glossary

Root Words

algesia (*sense of pain*)

angi/o (*vessel*)

arteri/o (*artery*)

cardiac arrest (*stopped heart*)

dactyl/o (*fingers*)

defibrillation (*heart shocked to a regular heartbeat*)

embolism (*obstruction of a blood vessel*)

embolus (*foreign particle in the bloodstream*)

esthesia (*feeling, sensation*)

fibrillation (*very fast,irregular heartbeat*)

myel/o (*spinal cord, bone marrow*)

phas/o (*speech*)

phleb/o (*vein*)

plas/o (*formation*)

thrombosis (*blood clot occluding a vessel*)

thrombus (*a blood clot*)

Prefixes

a-, an- (*absent, without*)

brady- (*slow*)

dys- (*bad, difficult, painful*)

macro- (*large*)

micro- (*small, very small*)

tachy- (*fast*)

Suffixes

poly- (*many*)

sym-, syn- (*together*)

-orrhexis (*rupture, bursting apart*)

-tripsy (*rubbing, crushing*)

-emia (*blood*)

Before you begin Chapter 6, take the time to complete the Review Sheet for Chapter 5. It will refresh your memory of the terms and word parts you studied. Find out how much you've learned.

The *heart* is the pump of the circulatory system. It is about the size of a fist. It's hollow and cone-shaped, with its apex at the bottom. The heart uses arteries to deliver oxygen-rich blood to the cells, tissues, and organs. Oxygen-depleted blood returns to the heart via the veins. The heart then pumps oxygen-deficient blood to the lungs where it becomes oxygen-enriched and returns to the heart for another circulatory round.

The *coronary arteries* are so named because they form an upside down "crown" on the surface of the heart. Both left and right arteries arise from small openings in the *aorta* just beyond the left side of the heart. The two main arteries form many branches and terminate in multitudes of tiny arteries that pass into the heart muscle and supply it with oxygen and nutrients.

Atherosclerotic plaque within the coronary artery may reduce blood flow and cause insufficient oxygen to reach the heart muscle.

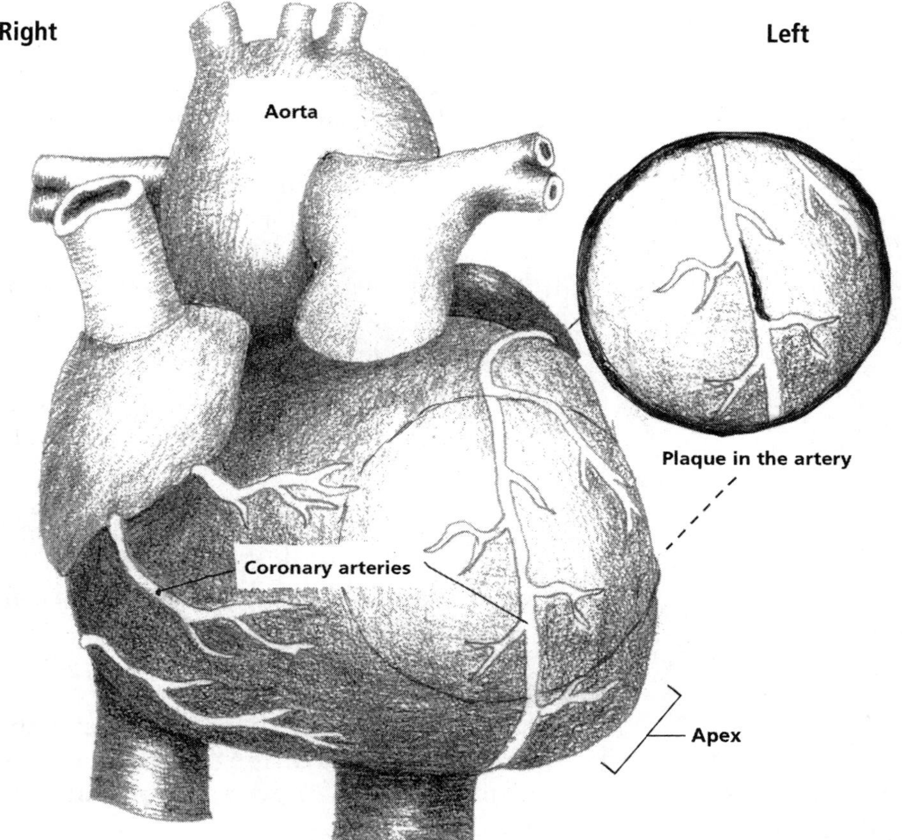

Figure 6.1. Coronary Arteries: Nourishment to the Heart

This condition often induces sharp, crushing chest pain. *Coronary thrombosis* means the coronary vessel may be occluded (closed off). Consequently, the cardiac muscle does not receive oxygen and can be severely damaged. *Fibrillation* (see below) may occur, and/or *cardiac arrest* may follow.

1.
Let's try something different. Some terms referring to abnormal conditions of the heart or blood vessels can be confusing. Read each definition carefully and select the terms that refer to a condition or procedure involving only the heart. Put an X in the box.

☐ (thrombus)
☒ (coronary thrombosis)

☐ (embolus)

☐ (embolism)
☒ cardiac arrest

☒ fibrillation
☒ defibrillation

☐ *Thrombus* is a circulating blood clot.
☐ *Coronary thrombosis* is a blood clot that occludes a coronary vessel of the heart and can cause an ischemic portion of the cardiac muscle.
☐ *Embolus* is a foreign or abnormal particle circulating in the blood, such as a bubble of air, a blood clot, or cholesterol plaque.
☐ *Embolism* is the sudden obstruction of a blood vessel by an embolus.
☐ *Cardiac arrest* is the complete cessation of heart function. (If the heartbeat cannot be restored, the patient dies.)
☐ *Fibrillation* means very fast and irregular heartbeat.
☐ *Defibrillation* means using an electrical impulse to shock the heart and bring about a regular heartbeat.

Now review the terms and their meanings again. This time *circle* each term that refers to a condition of the blood or blood vessels.

2.
Try these. A blood clot floating through the blood stream is known as a *thrombus*. When a blood clot occludes a vessel, the condition is called *thrombosis*. The part of the word meaning abnormal or diseased condition is ________________.

-osis

3.
Refer to the definitions in Frame 1. An embolus is any foreign or abnormal particle circulating in the blood, such as an air bubble, a cholesterol deposit, or even a blood clot. Embolism is the condition caused by an ________________.

embolus
em′ bō lus

A circulating blood clot is a ________________. But any foreign particle (including a blood clot) circulating through the bloodstream is an ________________.

thrombus
throm′ bus
embolus

4.
When a vessel is suddenly occluded by an embolus, the resulting condition is known as an ________________ism.

embol (ism)
em′ bō lizm

When a sudden vessel occlusion is caused by a thrombus, the resulting condition is a ________________osis.

thromb (osis)
throm bō′ sis

A blood clot occluding a coronary (heart) vessel is a condition called coronary ________________.

thrombosis

5.
Embolism is caused by an ________________.

embolus

Thrombosis is caused by a ________________.

thrombus

6.

coronary thrombosis

A sudden blocking or occlusion of the coronary vessel of the heart by a blood clot is a ________________ ________________.

7.

Cardiac fibrillation may result from coronary thrombosis. During this condition the heart beats 200 to 400 times a minute and is very irregular. If something is not done quickly, fibrillation will exhaust the heart and it will stop beating altogether.

An electrical spark can be utilized to shock the heart and bring about a slower and regular heartbeat, resulting in *de*fibrillation.

<u>defibrillation</u>
dē fib ri lā′ shun

Underline the term that indicates the better outcome:
cardiac arrest / defibrillation

8.

cardiac arrest

A very fast, irregular heartbeat, left unchecked, may lead to a complete cessation of heart functioning known as ________________ ________________.

9.

defibrillation

A very fast, irregular heartbeat is called fibrillation. Using an electrical spark to shock the heart and bring about a regular heartbeat is called ________________.

10.

Write the correct term for each of the following definitions:

thrombus — a blood clot floating through the bloodstream ________________

defibrillation — using an electrical impulse to shock the heart and restore a regular heartbeat ________________

cardiac arrest — complete cessation of heart functioning ________________ ________________

fibrillation — a very fast, irregular heartbeat ________________

embolism — sudden blocking or occlusion of a vessel by something that floated in the bloodstream ________________

coronary thrombosis — sudden blocking of the coronary vessel by a blood clot ________________ ________________

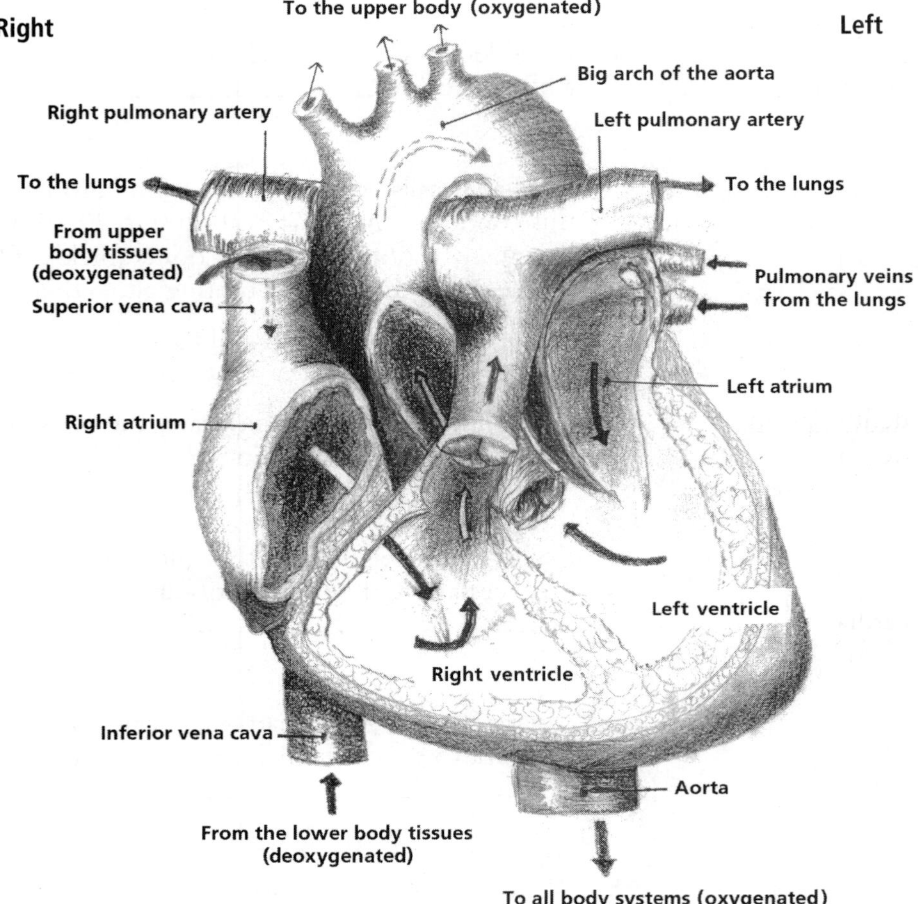

Figure 6.2 The Cardiovascular System

The *heart* is the muscular pump of the cardiovascular system. It pumps blood to the lungs and body systems and receives blood back for recirculation. Each day, the heart beats about 100,000 times at a rate of approximately 70 beats per minute.

The heart contains four cavities, or chambers: two on the right side (pulmonary heart), two on the left (systemic heart). Pulmonary circulation carries blood to and from the lungs. The systemic circulation supplies oxygen- and nutrient-rich blood to the body cells, tissues, and organs. After completing the systemic circuit, all blood returns to the heart through the two main veins, the *superior vena cava* and the *inferior vena cava*.

These vena cavae meet at the *right atrium*, a thin-walled chamber that serves as a collecting station. From the right atrium, the blood flows downward into the *right ventricle*, the smaller of the two muscular heart chambers. When the ventricle contracts, blood is forced upward, as in the illustration. It is pumped through the *right and left pulmonary arteries*, which lead to the two lungs. This begins the pulmonary circuit. Blood is pumped to the lungs for oxygenation, then returns to the heart for distribution to the body.

Blood from the lungs returns to the *left atrium* of the heart via the *pulmonary veins*. The veins are shown only on the left side of the heart; in the illustration they are hidden on the right side. From the left atrium (a collecting station) blood flows downward and enters the *left ventricle*, which is the larger of the two side-by-side muscular chambers. When the ventricles contract, simultaneously, the oxygenated blood is forced upward from the left ventricle through the big arch and into the aorta. From the aorta split all the arteries that perfuse the body tissues with oxygen and nutrients. Arteries arising from the aorta reach all parts of the head, upper extremities, thorax, abdomen, pelvic cavity, and lower extremities. After the blood nourishes the tissues, it returns to the heart to complete the circulation.

artery (arteri/o) vein (phleb/o)
vessel (angi/o) lung (pneumon/o)

abnormally slow

11.
Brady is used in words to mean abnormally slow.
Brady/cardia means __________ heart action.

brady/cardia
bradycardia
brad ē kär′ dē ə

12.
The term for abnormally slow heart action is
______________ / ________________.

abnormally fast or rapid heart action

13.
Tachy- is used in words to show the opposite of abnormally slow.
Thus tachy/cardia means ______________________________
____.

tachy/cardia
tachycardia
tak ə kär′ dē ə

14.
Write the medical term for an abnormally fast heartbeat:
______________ / ________________.

15.

Here's a quick review of what we have just covered. From List B select the best meaning for each term in List A. Write your choice in the space provided.

Answers	LIST A	LIST B
abnormally slow	brady- ________	foreign body in circulating blood
abnormally fast	tachy- ________	abnormally slow
foreign body in circulating blood	embolus ________	circulating blood clot
		abnormally fast
circulating blood clot	thrombus ________	very fast irregular heartbeat
very fast irregular heartbeat	fibrillation ________	

16.

heart

Arteries are vessels that carry oxygenated blood *away* from the heart. Veins are vessels that carry unoxygenated blood *back to* the ________________. This rule is only not true in cardiac circulation regarding oxygen status. Fetal circulation follows a different set of rules.

17.

a radiographic picture of the heart vessels (arteries and veins)

Note: Angi/o is the term used for vessels, whether the vessel is an artery or a vein.

What is a cardioangiogram? ________________________________

____

18.

arteries

phleb/o/scler/osis
phlebosclerosis
flēb′ ō skler ō′ sis

A combining form for vein is phleb/o. If arteriosclerosis is hardening of the ________________,

then hardening of veins is called

____________ / ______ / ______________ / ____________.
vein hardening condition

19.

phleb/otomy
phlebotomy
flē bot′ ō mē

phleb/itis
phlebitis
flē bī′ tis

Build a word meaning

incision into a vein (venisection or cut down)

______________ / ______________

inflammation of a vein

______________ / __________

	20.
clot	Thromb/o is the combining form that means clot. Thromb/o/angi/itis means inflammation of a vessel with formation of a __________________.
	21.
excision of a thrombus (clot)	Thromb/ectomy means ____.
	22.
inflammation of a vein with thrombus formation	Thromb/o/phleb/itis means ____.
	23.
thrombus	A synonym for clot is __________________.
	24.
thromb/osis thrombosis throm bō′ sis	Build a word meaning a condition caused by a clot ________________ / __________
thromb/o/cyte thrombocyte throm′ bō sīt	a cell that aids in clotting ________________ / ____ / __________
thromb/oid thromboid throm′ boid	resembling a clot ________________ / ________
	25.
	Let's review. Add the correct term to each of the definitions below.
Cardiac arrest	________________ ______________ is the complete cessation of heart function.
Coronary thrombosis	______________________ is a heart attack caused by a blood clot occluding the coronary blood vessel.
Defibrillation	__________________ is a procedure using an electrical spark to shock the heart and bring about a regular heartbeat.
Embolism	__________________ is the sudden obstruction of a blood vessel by an embolus.
Embolus	__________________ is a foreign or abnormal particle circulating in the bloodstream such as an air bubble, fat globule, or cholesterol plaque.

Fibrillation

________________ means a very fast (200–400 beats/min) and irregular heartbeat.

Thrombus

________________ is a blood clot in the bloodstream.

In this next section, you are taking on some new suffixes and prefixes.

26.
From the suggested answers select the meaning of each of the combining forms listed below.

SUGGESTED ANSWERS:

blood vessel	blood clot
artery	vein
lung(s)	

arteri/o ________________
thromb/o ________________
phleb/o ________________
angi/o ________________
pulmon/o ________________

It's time to take a short break.

27.
Try this one.

The suffix -orrhexis means rupture.

rupture of the bladder

Cyst/orrhexis means ________________
________________.

rupture of the small intestine

Enter/orrhexis means ________________
________________.

rupture of a blood vessel

Angi/orrhexis means ________________
________________.

cardi/orrhexis
cardiorrhexis
kär dē ō rek′ sis

phleb/orrhexis
phleborrhexis
flē bō rek′ sis

28.
Build a word meaning

rupture of the heart
__________ / ________________

rupture of a vein
__________ / ________________

29.
Here's a chance to use all the "orrh" suffixes with some combining forms to help you.

-orrhexis means rupture, bursting apart
-orrhagia means burst forth, hemorrhage
-orrhaphy means repair, suture together, close
-orrhea means flow, discharge

rhin/o saliping/o
cyst/o hepat/o

Build a medical term to satisfy each of the following definitions.

rupture of the (urinary) bladder
_______ / _______

cyst/orrhexis

hemorrhage from the liver
_______ / _______

hepat/orrhagia

flowing from the nose (runny nose)
_______ / _______

rhin/orrhea

suturing (or joining) the fallopian tubes
_______ / _______

salping/orrhaphy

What does herniorrhaphy mean? _______

suturing (or closing) a hernia

30.
Fill in the blank to complete these definitions

SUGGESTED ANSWERS:
-orrhagia -orrhaphy
-orrhea -orrhexis

_______ means repair, close, suture
_______ means burst forth, hemorrhage
_______ means discharge, flowing
_______ means rupture, bursting apart

-orrhaphy
-orrhagia
-orrhea
-orrhexis

31.
An- is a form of the prefix *a-* meaning without. *Esthesia* means feeling or sensation. Give the meaning of the following words:

anesthesia _______

a condition of being without feeling

anesthesiology ____

the study or science of removing feeling

instrument for measuring feeling or sensation

esthesiometer ____

abnormal sensitivity (to pain)

hyperesthesia ____

32.

Analyze the following words (you do the dividing):

an/esthesi/o/log/ist
an′ es thēz ē ol′ ō jist

anesthesiologist ____

hypo/esthes/ia
hī pō es thē′ zē ə

hypoesthesia ____

33.

without sensitivity to pain
an′ al jē′ zē ə

Algesia is a word meaning a sense of pain. What does analgesia mean? ____

34.

The prefixes *a-* and *an-* mean without. Examine the following two lists of words:

an/*a*lgesia	a/*b*iotic
an/*e*mia	a/*d*ermia
an/*e*ncephalus	a/*f*ebrile
an/*e*sthesia	a/*k*inesia
an/*o*nychia	a/*m*enia
an/*o*pia	a/*m*enorrhea
an/*u*ria	a/*p*nea
an/*u*resis	a/*s*epsis

a-

Draw a conclusion: When the word root begins with a consonant, use the prefix ________.

an-

When the word root begins with a vowel, use the prefix ________.

35.

Put the proper form of the prefix before each of the following roots and then write a meaning for each.

*an*emic—a condition of less blood

________emic ____

*a*stomia—without a mouth (congenital) | ________stomia ________________________________

*a*febrile—without fever | ________febrile ________________________________

*an*odontia— toothless | ________odontia ________________________________

36.
Here's some practice with other prefixes. *Phas/o* means speech. Write a meaning for each of the following:

speechless | aphasia ________________________________

abnormally fast speech | tachyphasia ________________________________

abnormally slow speech | bradyphasia ________________________________

pain or difficulty when speaking | dysphasia ________________________________

37.
Neur/o is used in words that refer to nerves. Neur/algia means ________________________________.

pain along the course of a nerve (or equivalent)

38.
Tripsis, from which we get trips/y, is a Greek word that means "rub" or "massage." Neur/o/trips/y means surgical crushing of a nerve. The word root for crushing (usually by rubbing or grinding) is ________________.

trips

Tripsis can be carried to the point of crushing or grinding. Surgical crushing of a nerve is called ____________ / ______ / ______________ / ______.

neur/o/trips/y
neurotripsy
nyo͞o′ rō trip sē

39.
In some cases of cholelithiasis, it may be necessary to crush calculi so they can pass from the gallbladder. A word meaning surgical crushing of gallstones is ____________ / ________ / _____ / ____________ / _____.

chole/lith/o/trips/y
cholelithotripsy
kō lē lith′ ō trip sē

40.
Myel/itis can mean either inflammation of bone marrow or inflammation of the spinal cord. From the definitions, you may conclude

bone marrow
spinal cord

that *myel* can be the word root for both ______________ and ______________.

41.
The suffix -*blast* means an immature cell (in the process of developing). In the term myel/o/blast, the word root myel refers to bone marrow. Write the meaning of myel/o/blast: ______________.

an immature bone marrow cell

In myel/o/cele, the word root refers to spinal cord. Write the meaning of myel/o/cele: ______________.

hernia of the spinal cord

42.
A medical term built on the word root myel may refer to different structures of the body. It may refer to either ______________ or ______________.

bone marrow or
spinal cord

43.
You have learned that dys- means pain, painful. But dys- is a prefix that also means bad (defective) or difficult. Try this.

Plasia means formation or change, in the sense of molding during the *growing years*. This kind of formation occurs naturally instead of being done by a plastic surgeon. Dys/plasia means ______________.

bad, defective (poor or abnormal formation)

44.
A/plasia means failure of an organ to develop properly. A term that means overgrowth or excessive development in the formative years is ______________ / ______________.

hyper/plasia
hyperplasia
hī′ per plā′ zha

45.
If overdevelopment is hyperplasia, underdevelopment is expressed as ______________ / ______________.

hypo/plasia
hypoplasia
hī′ pō plā′ zha

46.
Myel/o/dys/plasia means defective development of the spinal cord. What does chondr/o/dys/plasia mean? ______________

chondr/o/dys/plasia
chondrodysplasia
kon′ drō dis plā′ zhə
bad (defective) development of cartilage

oste/o/chondr/o/dys/plasia osteochondrodysplasia os′ tē ō kon′ drō dis plā′ zhə defective formation of bone and cartilage	47. Write the meaning of osteochondrodysplasia. ______

48.
Here's another quick review before moving on.

SUGGESTED ANSWERS:

-algesia	phas/o
-dys	plas/o
-tripsy	lith/o
	myel/o

Write the suffix or combining form that refers to each of the following words.

myel/o	spinal cord ______
phas/o	speech ______
-algesia	sensation of pain ______
lith/o	calculus ______
-tripsy	rubbing, crushing (procedure) ______
myel/o	bone marrow ______
dys-	painful, difficult, bad ______
plas/o	formation, development ______

49.
Explain the meaning of the following medical terms.

abnormally slow speech	bradyphasia ______
rubbing, crushing of a nerve	neurotripsy ______
incision to remove a gallstone	cholelithotomy ______
radiographic exam of the spinal cord	myelogram ______
bad development (formation) of cartilage	chondrodysplasia ______
lack of pain sensation	analgesia ______

50.

microns
mī′ krons

The *micron* (1/1000 mm) is a unit of measurement. Many cocci are 2 microns in diameter. A red blood cell is 7 ________ in diameter.

micr/o/meter
micrometer
mī krom′ ə ter

An instrument for measuring the diameter of something microscopic is a ________ / ________ / meter.

51.

large

On the other hand, *macr/o* is the opposite of micr/o. Macr/o is used in words to mean ________.

52.

a large immature cell visible by the naked eye

Things that are macr/o/scop/ic can be seen with the naked eye. Give a meaning for macroblast. ________

53.

macr/o/cephal/us
mak rō se fal′ us

An abnormally large head is ________ / ________ / ________ / ________.

macr/o/cyte

An abnormally large cell is a ________ / ________ / ________.

macr/o/cocc/us

A very large coccus is called a ________ / ________ / ________ / ________.

54.

In each case there is a condition of—

The suffix -ia indicates a condition. Pronounce each term and write a meaning.

abnormally large tongue
mak rō glos′ ē ə

macr/o/gloss/ia ________

abnormally large ear(s)
mak rō′ shē ə

macr/ot/ia ________

abnormally large nose
mak rō rin′ ē ə

macr/o/rhin/ia ________

abnormally large lips
mak rō kē′ lē ə

macr/o/cheil/ia ________

55.

dactyl
dak′ til

macr/o/dactyl/ia means abnormally large fingers or toes. The word root for fingers or toes is ________.

englarged digits, or another way of saying large fingers or toes	56. What does dactyl/o/megaly mean? ____________________
dactyl/o	57. A finger or toe is called a digit or dactyl. But the combining form for digit is ______________ / _____.
dactyl/itis dactylitis dak til ī′ tis	Build a term meaning inflammation of a digit ______________ / ____________
dactyl/o/spasm dactylospasm dak til′ ō spa zm	cramp or spasm of a digit ______________ / _____ / ______________
dactyl/o/gram dactylogram dak til′ ō gram	a fingerprint ______________ / _____ / ____________
abnormally large fingers and toes (digits)	58. Macr/o/dactyl/ia means ______________________________ ____.
fingers or toes (digits)	Poly/dactyl/ism means too many ____________________ ______________________________.
poly/ur/ia polyuria pol ē yer′ ē ə	59. *Poly-* is a prefix meaning too many or too much. Poly/ur/ia means excessive amount of urine. When a person drinks a lot of fluid, ____________ / _________ / _________ results.
polyneuritis pol ē nyo͞o rī′ tis	60. *Path* refers to disease. Poly/neur/o/path/y means disease of many nerves.
inflammation of many nerves	What does poly/neur/itis mean? ____________________ ____
inflammation of many joints	61. Write the meaning of the following: poly/arthr/itis ______________________________ ______________________________
pain in several nerves	poly/neur/algia ______________________________ ______________________________

	62.
syn/ergetic synergetic sin er je′ tik	Syn/ergetic means working together. Drugs that work together to increase the effects of one another are called ________ / ______________ drugs.
	63.
synergetic	Synergetic muscles are muscles that work together. It is on frequent occasions that a single movement requires multiple muscles working together. The function of these muscles is described as ________.
	64.
synergetic	APC tablets combine aspirin, phenacetin, and caffeine and are thought by some to be more effective for killing pain than aspirin alone. This is because *a*spirin, *p*henacetin, and *c*affeine are ____________ drugs.
	65.
a fused joint that moves as one	Syn/arthr/osis means an immovable joint; adjoining bones are fused together. When bones of a joint are fused so they all move as one, the condition is syn/arthr/osis. What does it mean? __________ ________________________________
syndactylism (syn underlined) synarthrosis (syn underlined)	Underline the part of the word that means joined together as one: syndactylism synarthrosis
	66.
a condition of two or more digits joined together as one	What does syn/dactyl/ism mean (-ism denotes a medical condition or disease)? ______________________________________
	67.
together or joined as one	*Syn-* and *sym-* are different forms of the same prefix: syn- and sym- mean ______________________________.
	68.
	Use the prefix sym- when the word root begins with the consonants b, m, or p; use syn- in all other cases. Write the prefix for each of the following:
syn-	______________ arthrosis
sym-	______________ metrical
sym-	______________ bolism
sym-	______________ physis
syn-	______________ drome

sym-	__________________ pathy
sym-	__________________ biosis

69.

Both syn- and sym- mean ________________________________; sym- is used when followed by the letters ________, ________, or ________; syn- is used in other medical words.

joined as one, together
b, m, p

70.

Time to review. Complete each brief definition. Refer to the suggested answers. Write your selection in the space provided.

SUGGESTED ANSWERS:

algesia	phas/o
brady	phleb/o
dactyl/o	plas/o
embolus	tachy
esthesia	

Answer	Definition
algesia	a sensation of pain __________________
phleb/o	veins __________________
embolus	foreign particle circulating in the blood __________________
esthesia	feeling, sensation __________________
phas/o	speech __________________
plas/o	formation, development __________________
dactyl/o	digits __________________
brady	abnormally slow __________________
tachy	abnormally fast __________________

71.

Try these.

SUGGESTED ANSWERS:

a-, an-	-orrhagia
dys-	-orrhaphy
macro-	-orrhexis
micro-	syn-, sym-
-orrhea	-tripsy

Answer	Definition
-orrhexis	rupture, burst apart __________________
syn-, sym-	together, as one __________________
dys-	defective, difficult, painful __________________
-orrhagia	hemorrhage, burst forth __________________

macro-	large ______
-tripsy	crushing, rubbing ______
micro-	microscopic, very small ______
-orrhea	flowing, discharge ______
a-, an-	without, absent ______
-orrhaphy	suturing (repair of) ______

Here are some suggestions:	72. In your own words, write the meaning for each of the following:
crushing of a nerve	neur/o/tripsy ______
without sensation of pain	an/esthesia ______
bad formation of the spinal cord	myel/o/dys/plasia ______
a condition of a blood clot in the coronary artery	coronary thrombosis ______ ______
pertaining to something too small to see with the naked eye	micro/scop/ic ______ ______
without speech, speechless	a/phasia ______
a condition of fingers joined together as one	syn/dactyl/ism ______
surgical repair of a hernia	herni/orrhaphy ______
hemorrhage of the liver	hepat/orrhagia ______
without, or absent, pain	an/algesia ______
complete cessation of heart function	cardiac arrest ______
electrical shock of the heart to restore regular rhythm	defibrillation ______ ______

ruptured blood vessel (vein)	phleb/orrhexis ______
abnormally slow heartbeat	brady/cardia ______

73.

Here are 32 medical terms for practicing your pronunciation. Say the term aloud and then say what it means. Then take the Chapter 6 Self-Test.

analgesia (an′ al jē′ zē ə)
anemia (an ē′ mē ə)
anesthesiologist (an′ es thē zē ol′ ō jist)
angiogram (an′ gē ō gram)
bradycardia (brad ē kär′ dē ə)
cardiorrhexis (kär dē ōr rek′ sis)
chondrodysplasia (kon′ drō dis plā′ zhə)
cystorrhexis (sis tō rek′ sis)
dactylogram (dak til′ ō gram)
dactylomegaly (dak′ til ō meg′ ə lē)
defibrillation (dē fib ri lā′ shun)
embolism (em′bō lizm)
embolus (em′ bō lus)
esthesiometer (es thē zē om′ ə ter)
hyperesthesia (hī′ per es thē′ zhə)
hypoesthesia (hī′ pō es thē′ zhə)
hypoplasia (hī′ pō plā′ zhə)
hysterorrhexis (his′ ter ō rek′ sis)
lithotripsy (lith′ ō trip sē)
macrocephalus (mak′ rō se fal′ us)
macrocheilia (mak′ rō kē′ lē ə)
macrotia (mak rō′ shē ə)
micrometer (mī krom′ ə ter)
neuromyelitis (nyo͞o′ rō mī il ī′ tis)
neurotripsy (nyo͞o′ rō trip sē)
phlebitis (flē bī′ tis)
polyarthritis (pol ē arth rī′ tis)
polyuria (pol ē yer′ ē ə)
syndactylism (sin dak′ til izm)
tachycardia (tak ə kär′ dē ə)
thrombosis (throm bō′ sis)
thrombus (throm′ bus)

Chapter 6 Self-Test

Part 1

From the list on the right, select the correct meaning for each of the following often used medical terms. Put the letter in the space provided.

______ 1. Lithotripsy
______ 2. Thrombosis
______ 3. Polyarthritis
______ 4. Anesthetist
______ 5. Synarthrosis
______ 6. Phlebitis
______ 7. Hysterorrhexis
______ 8. Dactylogram
______ 9. Analgesia
______ 10. Defibrillation
______ 11. Bradykinesia
______ 12. Neuromyelitis
______ 13. Macrocephalus
______ 14. Hypoesthesia
______ 15. Embolism
______ 16. Aphasia

a. Inflammation of a vein
b. Shocking the heart to restore a normal heartbeat
c. Obstruction of a blood vessel by an embolus
d. Abnormally enlarged head
e. Absence of pain
f. Inflammation of many joints
g. A specialist who removes all feeling or sensation
h. Crushing of a calculus
i. Bursting apart of the uterus
j. Fingerprint
k. Speechless
l. Clotted condition of a blood vessel
m. Inflammation of the nerves of the spinal cord
n. Less than normal sensation
o. Immovable joint, bones of a joint joined together as one
p. Abnormally slow movement

Part 2

Complete each of the medical terms on the right with the appropriate missing part or word.

1. Rupture (bursting apart) of the urinary bladder ______________________
2. Abnormally intense feeling or sensation ______________________
3. Foreign particle occluding a blood vessel ______________________ism
4. Rupture (bursting apart) of the heart ______________________
5. Abnormally large head ______________________
6. Inflammation of many nerves ______________________
7. Pain along the course of a nerve ______________________
8. A stopped heart ______________________(2 wds)
9. Abnormally large fingers ______________________
10. Foreign substance circulating in the bloodstream ______________________
11. Instrument for measuring feeling, sensation ______________________
12. A blood clot circulating in the bloodstream ______________________
13. Crushing destruction of a nerve ______________________
14. Absent the ability to speak, speechless ______________________
15. Fingers grown together as one ______________________
16. Abnormally fast heatbeat ______________________

ANSWERS

Part 1	*Part 2*
1. h.	1. Cystorrhexis
2. l.	2. Hyperesthesia
3. f.	3. Embolism
4. g.	4. Cardiorrhexis
5. o.	5. Macrocephalus
6. a.	6. Polyneuritis

7. i.	7. Neuralgia
8. j.	8. Cardiac arrest
9. e.	9. Dactylomegaly
10. b.	10. Embolus
11. p.	11. Esthesiometer
12. m.	12. Thrombus
13. d.	13. Neurotripsy
14. n.	14. Aphasia
15. c.	15. Syndactylism
16. k.	16. Tachycardia

7 Symptoms, Diagnoses, Treatments, Communication Qualifiers, and Statistics

In this chapter you will learn many terms related to signs and symptoms, diagnoses, treatments, and statistics. Some words will be familiar, but you'll use them in new ways.

Signs	**Qualifiers**	**Word Parts**
atrophy	acute	anti- (*against*)
edema	central	chlor/o (*green*)
hypertrophy	chronic	erythr/o (*red*)
pulse	generalized	melan/o (*black*)
respiration	localized	pyret/o (*fever*)
temperature	paroxysmal	xanth/o (*yellow*)
	peripheral	

Symptoms	**Treatments**	**Diagnoses**
anorexia	active	prodrome
dyspnea	palliative	prognosis
malaise	prophylactic	syndrome
nausea	systemic	
tinnitus		Statistics
vertigo		morbidity
		mortality

Be sure to complete the Chapter 6 Review Sheet before continuing.

Signs and Symptoms

1.

What are signs and symptoms? Signs are objective, able to be measured by an outside observer. Symptoms, on the other hand, are subjective, meaning the client experiences them. Symptoms are not readily available to an observer, and it is imperative that the individual give a complete description of the experience. An example of patients' signs and symptoms could be that they have a large laceration on their arm and they state that they are in pain. The laceration is the sign, and the pain they feel is the symptom. A patient experiences symptoms through one or more of the five organs of sense. Can you name them?

__________ __________ __________ __________ __________

sight
sound
smell
taste
feel

2.

Simply put, a sign or a symptom is evidence of either a normal or an abnormal body process. If it is something the client feels, tastes, hears, smells, or sees, it is a symptom. If it is something observed by the examiner, it is a sign. Sometimes signs and symptoms are reported together and may appear to be both. These reports can be divided into one or the other using the above definition. Let's practice:

Answer	SIGN	SYMPTOM	
sign	☐	☐	swelling of the wrist
symptom	☐	☐	ringing (tinkling sound) in the ear
symptom	☐	☐	sourness in the mouth
symptom	☐	☐	ammonia sensation in the nose
symptom	☐	☐	painful elbow
sign	☐	☐	blue discoloration around the eye
sign	☐	☐	very rapid breathing
symptom	☐	☐	pain in the heel
sign	☐	☐	fever
symptom	☐	☐	painful muscle spasm in the leg
sign	☐	☐	slow heartbeat
sign	☐	☐	pale complexion
sign	☐	☐	eyes closed, not responding to questions or poking

3.

An abnormality apparent to an examiner is called a ____________________.

sign

4.
Any change in body function or structure that the patient sees, hears, tastes, smells, or feels is called a ________________.

symptom

As you can see, most evidence of illness can be observed by someone other than the patient and may be experienced by the patient as well.

Vital Signs

5.
Vital means relating to life. A vital sign is evidence a patient is alive. Body temperature, pulse rate, rate of respiration, and blood pressure are vital signs because they provide continuous information about the essential processes of the body. If one of these signs is absent, the patient is dead (or in big trouble). Body temperature, pulse, respirations, and blood pressure are very important indicators and are called ________________.

vital signs

6.
Vital signs can be measured. Temperature (T) loosely refers to body heat above normal. Normal body temperature is 98.6°F. Body temperature increases in a hot environment and during physical exercise. Many diseases, serious and not serious, cause a patient's temperature to rise. Elevated body temperature is called *fever.* For adults, low fever is 99° to 101°F; moderate fever is 101° to 103°F; high fever is 103° to 105°F. Increased body temperature is the body's effort to make a bad environment for bacteria or viruses in order to kill them. A patient who is afebrile has a normal body temperature, which is approximately ________ °F.

98.6

7.
Pyro is a word root meaning fire or heat. (Remember the funeral pyres on which the Greeks and Romans burned their dead?) A pyromaniac has a fondness for watching things burn or starting ________________.

fires

8.
Pyret/o forms words meaning fever. A patient described as pyretic would have a temperature ________________ 98.6°F.
(above/below/same as)

above

9\.
Pyrexia means fever. Fever is one way the body shows something is wrong. Fever can be observed and measured; therefore, pyrexia is a ________________ of disease.
sign/symptom

sign

10\.
Hypo/thermia refers to body temperature below normal. A patient's temperature may be lowered safely to about 80° during surgery. This controlled procedure reduces the patient's need for oxygen and makes some surgical procedures safer. The patient's lower body temperature is called ________________.

hypothermia
hī pō ther′ mē ə

11\.
On the other hand, a person who falls through the ice on a pond in January will surely develop a life-threatening condition also called ________________.

hypothermia

12\.
Injury and dehydration can cause a patient's temperature to rise above 106°F. This life-threatening high temperature is known as ________________pyrexia.
(hyper/hypo)

hyper
hī per

13\.
In an earlier unit you learned that gen/o means to produce or originate. What does pyret/o/gen mean? ________________________________

that which produces fever

14\.
The measles virus produces fever. Therefore, the virus that causes measles is a ________________.

pyretogen
pī ret′ō jen

15\.
Pyret/ic means pertaining to fever. What does pyret/o/gen/ic mean? ________________________________

pertains to something that produces fever

16\.
Anti- means against. Aspirin is an anti/pyret/ic agent. What does antipyretic mean? ________________________________

an agent that works against fever

17.
Lysis means dissolution or reduction. What does pyret/o/lysis mean? ______________________

fever reduction

18.
A physician writes on a patient's chart, "The patient has a low-grade fever but is otherwise asymptomatic." What does asymptomatic mean? ______________________

without symptoms

19.
Now let's talk about another vital sign. Pulse (P) is a rhythmical throbbing of the arterial walls. This throbbing is produced when the heart contracts and forces an increased volume of blood into the vessels. After chasing your dog down the street, you would expect your pulse rate to ______________ (increase/decrease).

increase

20.
The normal pulse of an average adult is 70 to 80 beats per minute. Fever usually causes a patient's heart to beat more rapidly. When a patient's pulse is 100 beats per minute or higher the condition is known as ______________ (tachycardia/bradycardia).

tachycardia

On the other hand, a pulse less than 60 beats per minute indicates ______________.

bradycardia

21.
The patient usually does not feel a rapid, slow, or irregular pulse. However, a physician can observe and measure pulse rate; therefore, it is said to be a ______________ (sign/symptom).

sign

22.
Pulse rate depends on size, sex, age, and physical condition. It's higher in women than men. It's higher in children than adults. It is higher in infants than children. But we can say that a healthy adult has an average pulse of (check one)

☐ 30 to 50 beats per minute.
☐ 70 to 80 beats per minute.

70 to 80

23.
The pulse can be felt in many places: the umbilical stump in a newborn, a femoral artery in the groin, a pedal pulse in the foot, or the radial artery in the wrist. Although pulse is a simple measure, it provides important evidence about the life (and death) status of the patient. Therefore, it is considered a ________________.

vital sign

24.
Periphery means outer surface of the body. It is the part of the body away from the center. A pulse taken at the wrist or ankle is a ________________ pulse.
(central/peripheral)

peripheral
per i′ fer al

25.
A pulse taken near the center of the body, where the heart is, is a ________________ pulse.
(central/peripheral)

central

26.
A pulse taken with a stethoscope on the chest is a central pulse. Why? ________________

Because it is near the center of the body.

27.
What does peripheral mean? ________________

near the outer surface of the body

28.
Here's the third vital sign. Respiration (R) is breathing. Breathing is a function of the respiratory system. A breath draws in oxygen. The circulating blood carries the oxygen to the tissues and then returns carbon dioxide to the lungs. The lungs breathe out the waste products of carbon dioxide and water. The normal rate of respiration for an adult is 16 to 18 breaths per minute. A respiration rate of more than 25 breaths per minute is ________________ respiration.
(accelerated/decelerated)

accelerated

29.
Pne/o (pronounced nē o) means breath or breathing. Pne/o/dynamics means the mechanism of breathing. What does pne/o/meter mean? ________________

an instrument for measuring breathing

30.
Here's a rule that will help you pronounce words containing the root pne/o, pne/a. When pne/o begins the word, the letter "p" is silent. The letter "p" is pronounced when a prefix comes before it. Pronounce each of the following:

a/pnea	pronounce: ap′ nē ə
hyper/pnea	pronounce: hī perp′ nē ə
tachy/pnea	pronounce: tak ip nē′ ə
brady/pnea	pronounce: brad′ ip nē ə
pneumon/ia	pronounce: nū mon′ ē ə

very slow breathing

31.
Bradycardia means very slow heartbeat. What does brady/pnea mean? ______________________

disp′ nē ə
painful (bad) breathing

32.
Pronounce dys/pnea. What does it mean? ______________________
____

excessively rapid breathing
hī perp′ nē ə

33.
Hyperpyrexia means excessively high temperature (over 106°F). What does hyperpnea mean? ______________________
____

without breathing
ap′ nē ə

34.
A/symptomatic means without symptoms. What does a/pnea mean? ______________________

(Pronounce it.)

hyperpnea
hī perp′ nē ə

35.
Fever and disorders of the lungs or heart may accelerate respiration. Build a word that describes a respiration rate over 25 breaths per minute: ______________.

bradypnea
brad ip nē′ ə

36.
Very slow breathing of 8 to 9 breaths per minute occurs in serious illnesses like uremia, diabetic coma, and opium poisoning. Build a term that means very slow breathing: ______________.

37.
A foreboding irregular and unusual pattern of breathing is called Cheyne-Stokes respiration. (Pronounced *chain-stokes*. It's a condition

named after two physicians who first described it more than 150 years ago.) Respiration gradually increases in rapidity and volume until the rate reaches a climax (perhaps 60 to 80 breaths per minute). Then breathing subsides and ceases entirely for up to one minute—when respirations begin again. This condition is due to disturbance of the respiratory center in the brain. It is often a forerunner of death—but may last several months or days, or even disappear.

38.
Cheyne-Stokes respiration is cyclical. The phase of respiration, at 60 to 80 breaths per minute, is called hyperpnea. What term describes the period when all respiration ceases? ________________

apnea
ap′ nē ə

39.
In certain very serious illnesses, an irregular and arrythmic type of breathing may occur, characterized by both hyperpneic and apneic phases, often followed by death. It is called C________________-S________________ respiration. This condition is pronounced ________________ ________________.

Cheyne-Stokes
chain stokes

40.
The last vital sign is blood pressure. Blood pressure is part of the circulatory system and is how the body tries to balance the amount of blood delivered to the body. Blood pressure is measured in millimeters of mercury and measures the pressure inside the vascular system. Each blood pressure reading consists of a maximum pressure (systolic) and a minimum pressure (diastolic). These pressures can be altered if there is a problem with the functioning of the heart, if there is an abnormal amount of fluid in the circulatory system, if there is increased or decreased resistance inside the vessels, or if there is a change in blood viscosity. A normal blood pressure for an adult is 120/80, although there is a wide range of normal. A normotensive adult has the blood pressure of approximately ____________.

120/′0

41.
An elevated blood pressure would be classified as ________________.

hypertensive

A decreased blood pressure would be classified as ________________.

hypotensive

vital signs

temperature
pulse
respiration
blood pressure

42.
Something is very wrong with the body when a patient's respiration rate exceeds 25 breaths per minute. Respiration rate (R), fever (T), and a rapid pulse (P) are measurable signs of disease. They indicate the status of the whole body and are called __________ __________.

43.
The vital signs are T __________________, P __________________, R __________________, and B ____________ p______________.

44.
Let's review. Select the best meaning from column B for each brief definition in column A. Write your selection in the space provided.

COLUMN A	COLUMN B
bodily change a patient perceives ______________________	asymptomatic
sensory ways symptoms are perceived ______________________	vital signs
temperature, pulse, respiration, and blood pressure __________ __________	hyperpyrexia
elevated temperature, fever ______________________	hypothermia
subnormal body temperature ______________________	hypotension
temperature over 106°F ______________________	hypertension
something that produces fever ______________________	pyretogen
reduction, dissolution of fever ______________________	pyrteolysis
lack of symptoms ______________________	pyrexia
above normal blood pressure ______________________	see, hear, smell, taste, feel
below normal blood pressure ______________________	symptom

symptom
see, hear, smell, taste, feel

vital signs
pyrexia
pī rek′ sē ə
hypothermia
hī pō ther′ mē ə
hyperpyrexia
hī per pī rek′ se ə
pyretogen
pī ret′ ō gen
pyretolysis
pī ret ō lī′ sis
asymptomatic
ā simp tō mat′ ik

hypertension

hypotension

45.
Now try these.

Answers	COLUMN A	COLUMN B
		apnea
pulse	throbbing of an artery in time with the heartbeat ____________	bradypnea
peripheral	pulse taken at the surface of the body ____________	Cheyne-Stokes respiration
pne/o, pne/a	two combining forms for breath, breathing ____________ or ____________	dyspnea
bradypnea	very slow breathing ____________	hyperpnea
dyspnea	difficult breathing ____________	peripheral
hyperpnea	excessively fast breathing ____________	pne/o, pne/a
respiration	another word for breathing ____________	pulse
apnea	respiratory arrest, not breathing ____________	respiration
Cheyne-Stokes respiration	breathing that reaches a climax, then ceases before beginning again ____________-____________ ____________	

Color and Other Signs

46.
Color and changes in color of various parts of the body also tell the physician a lot about the patient's condition. For example, tissue that is black may be dead tissue, red tissue may indicate infection, blue tissue may have too little oxygen, white tissue may have too little circulating blood; yellow or green discharge could indicate infection, or yellow tissue could indicate liver disfunction. There are many other things color can tell us. Use the information here to build words involving color.

leuk/o	white
melan/o	black
erythr/o	red
cyan/o	blue
chlor/o	green
xanth/o	yellow

	47.
xanth/opsia zan thop′ sē ə	Cyan/opia means blue vision. Form a word meaning yellow vision ____________________/opsia
chlor/opia klor ō′ pē ə	green vision ____________________/opia
	48.
erythr/o/derma e rith′ rō der′ mä	Cyan/o/derma means blue skin. Build a word meaning red skin ______________ / _____ / ____________
melan/o/derma mel′ a nō der′ mä	black (discolored) skin ____________________ (You draw the lines.)
	49.
	Write a meaning for each of the following:
green (plant) cell white (blood) cell red (blood) cell	chlor/o/cyte ________________________________. leuk/o/cyte ________________________________. erythr/o/cyte ________________________________.
	50.
	-blast means immature cell. Build a word meaning an immature cell of the following colors:
melan/o/blast mel′ a nō blast	immature black cell ______________ / _____ / ______________ black immature cell
erythr/o/blast e rith′ rō blast	immature red cell ________________ / _____ / ____________
	51.
	Melan/osis means a condition of black pigmentation. Carcinoma is a malignant tumor.
a black-pigmented malignant tumor	What is a melanocarcinoma? ________________________________ __________________________
	52.
melanocarcinoma mel′ a nō kär si nō′ mä	Whenever a hairless mole on the skin turns black and grows larger, a physician should be consulted because there is a risk of black mole cancer, or ________________________.
	53.
green red yellow white	Chlor/o means ____________________. Erythr/o means ____________________. Xanth/o means ____________________. Leuk/o means ____________________.

Qualifiers

54.
In medical terminology we often use qualifiers. These are adjectives or adverbs that when used with another word make the meaning of that term more specific. Here are a few frequently used qualifiers. *Local* means a small area or part of the body. *General* means involving the whole body or many different areas or parts of the body at the same time.

55.
Anesthesia may be considered either local or general. Before extracting a tooth, the dentist injects Novocain to prevent pain. Novocaine is a ____________________ anesthetic.
(local/general)

local

56.
On the other hand, laughing gas, which puts the patient to sleep, is a ____________________ anesthetic.
(local/general)

general

57.
When referring to a disease process, the words can be used in the form of localized or generalized. Use either localized or generalized as a label for each of the following.

skin rash around the neck and ears
____

localized

measles macules from stem to stern
____

generalized

acne all over the face
____

localized

second-degree scalding burn over the belly and upper thigh
____

localized (two places)

reddish-purple spots over the trunk of the body and wherever clothing covers the skin
____

generalized

58.
A localized condition means it is ______________________________
____.

limited to a small area or part of the body

involving the whole body or many areas at the same time

When a condition is generalized, it means it is ________________________________.

59.

general

Systemic means pertaining to all body systems, or the whole body rather than one of its parts. It is another word for ____________ (local/general).

60.

systemic
sis tem′ ik
or general

An antihistamine tablet helps a patient breathe more easily by drying up mucous membranes inside the nose and sinuses. An antihistamine also dries up mucous membranes that line all body cavities. We say it has a ______________ effect.

Other Signs

Besides observing color and color changes, a physician inspects the patient carefully for signs and symptoms that will aid in learning about a patient's disease. Here are some observable changes in the body.

61.

fluid

Edema refers to fluid accumulation in the tissues. It is a condition in which body tissues accumulate excessive ____________.

62.

the whole body

Fluid in the tissues may be local or general. Localized edema involves a small area of the body; generalized edema involves ______________________________.

63.

edema
e dē′ ma

A bee sting produces an accumulation of fluid in the tissues at the bite site. This is called localized ______________.

64.

generalized edema

Heart failure causes severe disturbance of the body's water balance mechanisms. Excessive fluid may accumulate in the lungs, legs, and abdomen. This condition is called ____________________ (localized/generalized) (two words).

65.

edema

Excessive accumulation of fluid in the body tissues is called ____________.

66.
Atrophy is another observable sign of disease. It means a wasting away or shrinking of tissues, an organ, or the whole body. Underline the word root meaning development.

A<u>trophy</u>
at′ rō fē

Atrophy

What does hyper/troph/y mean?

overdevelopment

____

67.
It's time to review. Select the best meaning from Column B for each color listed in Column A. Write your selection in the space provided.

Answer	COLUMN A	COLUMN B
erythr/o	red ____________	cyan/o
leuk/o	white ____________	chlor/o
cyan/o	blue ____________	erythr/o
chlor/o	green ____________	melan/o
xanth/o	yellow ____________	leuk/o
melan/o	black ____________	xanth/o

68.
Select a suggested answer to complete each of the following definitions.

SUGGESTED ANSWERS:

edema	local
generalized	systemic
hypertrophy	atrophy

generalized — (a) ____________ means pertaining to the whole body or many areas at the same time.

systemic — (b) Another term meaning the same as (a) above is ____________.

local — (c) An injection of anesthetic under the skin of the forearm to remove a mole is described as a ____________ anesthetic.

edema — (d) Accumulated excess fluid in the tissues of the lower extremities may be a condition of ____________.

atrophy — (e) A wasting away or shrinking of tissues of an organ or a body part is described as ____________.

hypertrophy — (f) ____________ is the term that describes the opposite of (e) above.

Subjective Symptoms

Objective *signs* such as T, P, R, and BP are *signs* of primary importance in the investigation of an illness. However, the patient's own concerns and impressions also provide valuable information. Changes in the body not apparent to an observer but experienced by the patient are called *symptoms*.

69.
Nausea means sickness of the stomach with a desire to vomit. Since it is an internal feeling evident only to the patient, we call it a ________________.

symptom

70.
Pain, noxious odors, fevers, and some drugs may cause a sickness of the stomach with a desire to vomit, which is called ____________.

nausea
naw′ zē ə

71.
Mal de mer is the French term meaning motion sickness. It is another way to describe the sick feeling of ____________.

nausea

72.
Emesis means vomitus—that which is vomited. An irritation of the vomiting center in the brain produces nausea. As a result, the patient ejects the stomach contents through the mouth. The product of vomiting is ______________________________.

emesis (or vomitus)
em′ e sis

73.
Food poisoning, drugs, and fevers can irritate the vomiting center and thus induce ________________. The product of vomiting is ____________.

vomiting
emesis

74.
Chol/emesis means bile in the vomitus. What does hemat/emesis mean? ____

blood in the vomitus

75.
In an emergency, there are two quick ways to empty the stomach of its contents: (a) use a tube to "pump" the stomach, or (b) give the patient an emetic. What is an emetic? ________________
____

something that induces vomiting

(nausea) The patient feels the sensation (not observable).	76. *Nausea* usually precedes *emesis*. Circle the term that is a subjective symptom. Why? ______
malaise	77. In a wide variety of illnesses, two symptoms often occur together. We'll take them one at a time. *Malaise* is a French word literally meaning ill at ease. Underline the part of the word meaning ill.
malaise ma lī′z	78. A patient with infectious mononucleosis may experience a vague sensation of not feeling well, or feeling ill at ease. The symptom is called ______.
the vague sensation of not feeling well	79. Malaise is a symptom because the physician cannot observe malaise and does not experience the patient's sensation. Describe malaise. ______
loss of appetite an o rek′ sē ə	80. Orexia means appetite. What does an/orexia mean? ______
pertaining to something that produces or stimulates an appetite	81. Orexi/mania means an abnormal desire (madness) for food or an uncontrollable appetite. What does orexi/genic mean? ______
orexigenic ō reks i gen′ ik	82. Food that smells good and is appealing to the eye stimulates appetite. We may describe this food and its presentation as ______.
anorexia an o rek′ sē ə	83. Along with malaise, loss of appetite is a very common symptom in many diseases. Write the term for loss of appetite: ______.

84.
Complete each of the following definitions:

malaise	A vague sensation of not feeling well is ________________.
nausea	Sickness of the stomach with a desire to vomit is ________________.
emesis	Another word for vomitus is ________________.
pyrexia	Elevated body temperature is ________________.
anorexia	Loss of appetite is ________________.

85.
A patient with an infection may experience a vague sensation of not feeling well. A patient with a fever may not have an appetite. When a fever and infection occur at the same time, the patient usually reports these two very subjective symptoms. What are they? ________________ and ________________

malaise
anorexia

86.
Anorexia and malaise are purely subjective symptoms. What does that mean? ____

The patient experiences the sensation.

87.
Vertigo means a turning around. The patient experiences the sensation of turning around in space or having objects move about him.

88.
Vertigo is *not* dizziness, faintness, or lightheadedness. However, the patient may have difficulty maintaining equilibrium, and may describe a sensation of spinning or ________________________ in space.

turning around

89.
An infection in the middle ear can cause a patient to experience the sensation of turning around in space or of objects moving about her. This ________________ (sign/symptom) is known as ________________.

symptom
vertigo
ver′ ti gō

90.
Tinnitus is a jingling, or tinkling, sound in the ear. It is often called ringing in the ear.

Toxicity or sensitivity to a drug like aspirin can cause ringing in the ear. Write the medical term for tinkling sound in the ear: ________________.

tinnitus
ti nī′ tus

91.

Ménière's syndrome (pronounce ma nē ars′) is a recurrent and usually progressive group of symptoms including hearing loss, ringing in the ears, a sensation of fullness or pressure in the ears, and a turning around in space.

Answer	
tinnitus	The term for ringing in the ears is ________________.
vertigo	The sensation of turning about in space is ________________.

92.

Try these and see how much you've learned. Select the best word from the suggested answers.

SUGGESTED ANSWERS:

erythroderma leukocyte
melanoblast cyanemia
chlorocyte xanthemia

Answer	
chlorocyte	green (plant) cell ________________
xanthemia	yellowish blood ________________
melanoblast	black (dark) immature cell ________________
erythroderma	reddened skin ________________
leukocyte	white blood cell ________________
cyanemia	blue-bloodedness ________________

93.

Now try these qualifiers.

hypertrophia atrophy
general systemic
local

Answer	
general or systemic	pertaining to the entire body ________________
hypertrophia	overdevelopment ________________
local	pertaining to a small area, or one part ________________
systemic	pertaining to all body systems ________________
atrophy	a wasting away, underdevelopment ________________

94.

Here are some objective symptoms.

tinnitus malaise
emesis nausea
vertigo anorexia

vertigo	a sensation of turning around in space ______
nausea	seasickness; inclined to vomit ______
emesis	another word for vomitus ______
tinnitus	ringing in the ears ______
malaise	a vague sensation of not feeling well ______
anorexia	loss of appetite ______

Describing Illness

95.
A diagnosis is an identification of an illness. It requires scientific and skillful methods to establish the cause and nature of a sick person's disease. A diagnosis is arrived at by evaluating (a) the history of the person's disease, (b) the signs and symptoms present, (c) laboratory data, and (d) special tests such as X rays and electrocardiograms.

96.
In your English dictionary, you'll find words beginning with gnos. They come from the Greek word *gnosis,* meaning knowledge. *Dia* means through. Therefore, dia/gnosis literally means ______.

knowing through

97.
Diagnosing an illness means studying it through its signs and symptoms and other available information. When a patient reports chills, feels hot, and has a runny nose, the physician may identify the patient's illness as a head cold. This conclusion would be the ______.

diagnosis
dī ag nō′ sis

98.
A patient complains of pain in her arm after falling off her horse. An X ray shows a broken bone in her forearm. With this information from an X ray, the physician arrives at a ______.

diagnosis

99.
What do you think hemodiagnosis means? ______

identification of a patient's illness through blood (studies)

100.
Many diseases are complex, so establishing the cause and nature of a sick person's disease requires skill and scientific methods. Which of the following might a physician use to help identify an illness? Check one or more.

(all are relevant)

- ☐ personal and family history
- ☐ signs and symptoms
- ☐ laboratory data
- ☐ special tests, such as an X ray or ECG

101.
If an obstetrician is one who is skilled in delivering babies, what is a diagnostician? ______________________________

one who is skilled in making diagnoses

102.
The prefix pro- means before, or in front of. What do you think is the meaning of prognosis? ______________________________

Here's our suggestion: to predict the patient's illness (its course and outcome)

103.
Acute leukemia often may be fatal within three months. Prediction of the course and outcome of this disease is called a ____________.

prognosis
prog nō′ sis

104.
What does prognosticate mean? ______________________________

to tell what the course and likely outcome of the disease will be

105.
A prognosis predicts the course and outcome of a disease. Select a term that best fits each outcome described.

favorable unfavorable guarded

Expect the patient to die in 3 to 6 months: ____________.
Recovery will be easy after surgery: ____________.
Recovery will be long and difficult: ____________.

unfavorable
favorable
guarded

106.
A patient who has little chance of recovering from his disease is said to have an (two words) ____________ ____________.
unfavorable/favorable predicted outcome

unfavorable prognosis

Answer	Frame
diagnosis	107. When a physician has identified the patient's illness, the physician has made a ________________.
prognosis	108. Prediction of the course and outcome of the disease is a ________________.
paroxysm par′ ok sizm and paroxysmal par ok siz′ mal	109. A diagnosis may specify that the disease is acute, chronic, or paroxysmal. *Acute* means sharp, severe, having a rapid onset and a short course, not chronic. *Chronic* means long, drawn-out. A chronic disease is not acute. *Paroxysmal* is from the Greek word *paroxysm*. It means a sudden periodic attack or recurrence of symptoms of disease, a fit or convulsion of any kind.
chronic kron′ ik	110. Diabetes is a disease that has a long, drawn-out course. Therefore, diabetes is a ________________ (acute/chronic/paroxysmal) disease.
paroxysmal par ok sis′ mal	111. Epilepsy is characterized by a sudden onset of symptoms that recur periodically. Therefore, epilepsy is a ________________ (acute/chronic/paroxysmal) illness.
sudden recurring episode of difficult breathing	112. Dys/pnea means difficult breathing. Paroxysmal dyspnea is another way to describe asthma. Explain paroxysmal dyspnea. ________________
stomach rapid severe short	113. Gastritis may be acute or chronic. Acute gastritis means inflammation of the ________________. Its onset is ________________ (rapid/slow), the pain in the belly is ________________ (mild/severe), and the illness lasts a ________________ (short/long) time.

114.
A patient has a sudden onset of fast heart rate—in excess of 200 beats per minute—and then abruptly the heart rate returns to normal. This has occurred before. The diagnosis would be

paroxysmal tachy/cardia

__________ (acute/chronic/paroxysmal) __________ (rapid) / __________ (heart).

115.
Arteriosclerotic heart disease (ASHD) has a very slow onset. Symptoms may be mild and last a lifetime. ASHD is a/an __________ condition.

chronic

116.
Inflammatory conditions may be either acute or chronic. Acute tendonitis means the tendon becomes red, hot, and very painful in a short period of time. It returns to normal after a day or two of treatment.

Describe chronic tendonitis: ____.

inflammation that has a slow onset (may be mild) and lasts a long time

117.
A fit or convulsion is a/an __________.

paroxysm
par′ ok sizm

A long, drawn-out disease is described as __________.

chronic

Sharp, severe symptoms, over a short course, describe a/an __________ disease.

acute

118.
Poly- is a prefix meaning many or much; excessive. Explain each of the following:

Acute polyneuritis means ____.

an inflammation of many nerves, a rapid onset; very painful, short duration

Chronic polyarthritis means ____.

an inflammation of many joints that starts slowly and lasts a long time

Polydactylism means ____.

a condition of having supernumerary fingers (or toes)

119.
Syndrome is a group of signs and symptoms that occur together and thus characterize a specific disease.

a group of signs and symptoms running along together

Syn means together; *drome* means running along. Therefore, syndrome literally means ____.

120.
For example, Korsakoff's syndrome is a psychosis, ordinarily due to chronic alcoholism. It is characterized by polyneuritis, disorientation, insomnia, muttering delirium, hallucinations, and a bilateral wrist or foot drop. Korsakoff's syndrome is characterized by this group of signs and symptoms that occur ________________.

together

121.
A syndrome is a variety of signs and symptoms occurring together. When signs and symptoms run along together, they present a complete picture of the disease. This is known as a ________________.

syndrome
sin′ drōm

122.
Alcoholism produces a characteristic group of signs and symptoms called Korsakoff's syndrome. From the name we know that a variety of ____________ and ____________ occur ______________.

signs
symptoms
together

123.
A group of symptoms occurring together characterize a specific disease. We call this group of symptoms a ________________.

syndrome

124.
Recurrent (and usually progressive) hearing loss, tinnitus, vertigo, and a sensation of fullness in the ears is known as Ménière's ________________.

syndrome

Explain why: ____.

The symptoms run along together.

125.
Pro/drome means running before (a disease). A symptom or group of symptoms that occur a few hours or a few days before the onset of the disease are called prodromal symptoms. These early signals are called its ________________.

prodrome
prō′ drom

126.

The prodromal phase of a disease is the interval between the earliest symptoms and the appearance of a rash or fever. These symptoms occur ________________ (before/after) the onset of the disease.

before

127.

Sneezing that comes before the chills and fever of a common cold are the ________________ symptoms of the cold.

prodromal

128.

Malaise, anorexia, and sore throat occur one to four days before the fever and rash of measles appear. This early stage of the disease is called the ________________ phase.

prodromal
prō drō′ mal

129.

It's time to review what you just covered. From the suggested answers, select the best term for each brief definition.

asymptomatic	acute
prognosis	prodromal
chronic	diagnose
syndrome	paroxysm

to identify an illness ________________ — diagnose

a sudden, recurrent attack ________________ — paroxysm

pertaining to severe symptoms and rapid onset ________________ — acute

prediction of course and outcome of illness ________________ — prognosis

symptoms occurring together as a disease ________________ — syndrome

relating to symptom-free ________________ — asymptomatic

pertaining to a long, drawn-out illness ________________ — chronic

earliest phase of signals and symptoms occurring before the onset of the fever or rash associated with a disease ________________ — prodromal

130.

Using the standard method of investigation called the head-to-toe assessment, a health care provider gathers information about a patient's illness in order to learn the cause and nature of a sick person's disease. Identification of the illness is called a ________________.

diagnosis

Treatment

Treatment is the medical, surgical, or psychiatric management of a patient's illness. Although there are many different kinds of treatments, we're covering only a few of the most common.

131.

Active treatment aims for a cure. A patient suffering from appendicitis expects to be cured after an appendectomy. Since surgery removes the patient's appendix and usually cures the patient's disease, it is an __________ treatment.

active

132.

An antibiotic attacks the bacteria causing peritonitis. Therefore, antibiotic therapy is considered an __________ treatment.

active

133.

Systemic treatment attacks constitutional signs and symptoms such as pyrexia, shock, and pain. Treatment directed toward control of these life-threatening signs is called __________ treatment.

systemic
sis tem′ ik

134.

Giving a patient morphine for pain is a systemic treatment that aims to relieve a __________ sign or symptom.

life-threatening or constitutional

135.

Hyperpyrexia is a constitutional sign. Placing a hyperpyrexic child in a basin of ice water reduces the whole body temperature and is therefore a __________ treatment.

systemic

136.

Palliative treatment relieves bothersome symptoms and makes a patient comfortable. Very little the physician can do alters the course of poison ivy dermatitis. The physician may suggest calamine lotion to reduce itching and burning, and therefore, calamine is called a __________ treatment.

palliative
pal′ ē a tiv

137.

Prophylaxis is a treatment modality that focuses on prevention of disease. Your dentist aims to prevent dental cavities by applying flouride solution to your teeth. Flouride application is called a __________ treatment.

prophylactic
prō fi lak′ tic

138.
Whether active, symptomatic, palliative, or prophylactic, things the physician does or prescribes to manage a patient's illness are called ____________________.

treatments

139.
Palliative treatment addresses a patient's comfort rather than attempting to cure the disease. The purpose of this kind of treatment is to ____.

relieve symptoms

140.
Active treatment squarely addresses the patient's pathological condition. The physician elects an active treatment modality when a remedy or therapy will ________________ the disease.

cure
kyo͞or

141.
Shock, pyrexia, and pain are indications of disease that if not treated could have very serious consequences. Systemic treatment is directed toward very serious constitutional signs of illness that may be ________________________.

life-threatening

142.
From the terms listed, select one that best fits each description.

active	palliative
prophylactic	systemic

treatment of constitutional symptoms ____________________

treatment directed specifically toward a cure ____________________

treatment to relieve discomfort ____________________

treatment aimed at preventing disease ____________________

systemic
active
palliative
prophylactic

143.
There are many remedies and therapies a physician may use to treat a patient's illness. Here are a few of the major classes for you to investigate. Look up *therapy* and see if you can define the words below.

pharmacotherapy	radiotherapy
physical therapy	electroshock therapy
chemotherapy	psychotherapy

Statistics

In medicine and health care, many people keep score. The Department of Health and Human Services (HHS) of the U.S. government and the World Health Organization (WHO) of the United Nations publish statistics showing how many people are affected by certain diseases and how many people die of their illnesses. In order to understand the statistics, there are two important terms to know: *morbidity* and *mortality*.

144.

Morbidity means a diseased state. A statistic that reports, "50 cases of measles per 10,000 people living in the United States last year" is called a ______________________ rate.

morbidity (or sickness)
mor bid′ i tē

145.

Mortality means the state of being mortal and, therefore, subject to death. In other words, mortality is a statistic that reports the ______________________ rate.

mortality (or death)
mor tal′ i tē

146.

Which of the following examples expresses a mortality rate? Check each correct example.

- □ In 2008, 37,261 people were killed in automobile accidents on U.S. highways.
- □ In 2003–2004, malaria accounted for 52–78% of deaths in Ethiopia.
- □ Nearly 22,000 U.S. deaths are estimated in 2009 from leukemia.

(all three are mortality statistics)

147.

The mortality rate is the same as saying the ____________ rate.

death

148.

The morbidity rate is expressed as the number of cases of a specific disease found in a specific unit of population during a specific period of time. It shows the rate of ______________________.

sickness or disease

149.

Which of the following examples is a morbidity rate? Check each correct example.

(the top one shows a morbidity rate)

- ☐ Between 2005 and 2007 there were less than 15 new cases of tuberculosis reported for every 100,000 people living in the United States.
- ☐ In 2009, there were 10.9 deaths from suicide for every 10,000 people in the United States.

150.
A statistic that reports the number of cases of a disease in a specific population for a specific period of time is called ________________ ________________.

morbidity rate

151.
A statistic that reports the death rate is called ________________ ________________.

mortality rate

152.
What is the difference between a morbidity and a mortality statistic?
____
____
____

Morbidity refers to the rate of illness; mortality refers to the death rate.

153.
In this chapter you worked with many new terms and learned to use some familiar words in new ways. Fifty of these words are listed here for you to practice your pronunciation and to review their meanings. Pronounce each term, think about its meaning, and then take the Chapter 7 Self-Test.

acute (a kūt′)
anorexia (an o rek′ sē ə)
antipyretic (an tē pī ret′ ik)
asymptomatic (ā simp tō mat′ ik)
atrophy (at′ rō fē)
bradypnea (brad′ ip nē ə)
central (sen′ trul)
Cheyne-Stokes respiration (ch1n-stōks)
chlorocyte (klor′ ō sīt)
chronic (kron′ ik)
cyanoderma (sī ə nō der′ mä)
diagnosis (dī ag nō′ sis)
dyspnea (disp′ nē ə)
edema (e dē′ mä)
emesis (em′ ə sis)
erythremia (er i thrē′ mē ə)
generalized
hematemesis (hē mä tem′ ə sis)
hyperpnea (h perp′ nē ə)
hyperpyrexia (hī per pī rek′ sē ə)
hypothermia (hī pō ther′ mē ə)
leukocyte (lo͞o′ kō sīt)
localized
malaise (mä lāz′)
melanocarcinoma (mel′ ə nō kär sin ō′ mä)
morbidity (mor bid′ i tē)

mortality (mor tal′ i tē)
nausea (naw′ zē ə)
palliative (pal′ ē ə tiv)
paroxysmal (par ok sis′ mal)
peripheral (per i′ fer al)
pneometer (nē om′ ə ter)
polyarthritis (pol′ ē arth rī′ tis)
prodromal (prō drō′ mal)
prognosis (prog nō′ sis)
prophylactic (prō fi lak′ tic)
pulse (puls)
pyretolysis (pī ret ō lī′ sis)
pyrexia (pī rek′ sē ə)
respiration
symptom
symptomatic
syndrome (sin′ drōm)
systemic
tachypnea (tak ip nē′ ə)
temperature
tinnitus (ti nī′ tus)
vertigo (ver′ ti gō)
vital signs
xanthopsia (zan thop′ sē ə)

Chapter 7: Self-Test

Part 1

From the list on the right, select the correct meaning for each of the following medical terms.

______	1. Diagnosis	a.	Pertaining to the whole body, all systems
______	2. Systemic	b.	Very fast breathing
______	3. Morbidity	c.	Identification of an illness
______	4. Pyretolysis	d.	Fluid in the tissues
______	5. Edema	e.	Pertaining to disease rate statistic
______	6. Generalized	f.	Temperature, pulse, and respiration
______	7. Anorexia	g.	Reduction of fever
______	8. Vertigo	h.	A sickness of the stomach; desire to vomit
______	9. Hyperpnea	i.	Pertaining to the whole body, many different parts at the same time
______	10. Malaise		
______	11. Paroxysm	j.	Wasting away, or underdevelopment
______	12. Vital signs	k.	Loss of appetite
______	13. Syndrome	l.	Sensation of turning around in space
______	14. Nausea	m.	Vague sensation of not feeling well
______	15. Atrophy	n.	Pertaining to sudden periodic attack
		o.	Symptoms occurring together

Part 2

Complete each of the medical terms on the right with the appropriate missing part. Some terms are missing all parts!

1. Ringing in the ear ____________
2. Artery throbbing in time with the heartbeat ____________
3. Respiratory arrest, not breathing ____________
4. Outside surface of the body ____________
5. Pertaining to preventing disease ____________
6. Sudden recurring attack ____________
7. Symptom-free ____________
8. Breathing that reaches a climax, then ceases before beginning again C____________-S____________ respiration
9. Pertaining to relieving symptoms but not the disease ____________
10. Patient perceives change in body or functions ____________
11. Prediction of course and outcome of a disease ____________
12. Pertaining to severe symptoms, rapid onset, short course ____________
13. Reddened skin ____________
14. Subnormal body temperature under 90°F ____________
15. Feverishness ____________

ANSWERS

Part 1	*Part 2*
1. c	1. Tinnitus
2. a	2. Pulse
3. e	3. Apnea

4. g	4. Peripheral
5. d	5. Prophylactic
6. i	6. Paroxysm
7. k	7. Asymptomatic
8. l	8. Cheyne-Stokes respiration
9. b	9. Palliative
10. m	10. Symptom
11. n	11. Prognosis
12. f	12. Acute
13. o	13. Erythroderma
14. h	14. Hypothermia
15. j	15. Pyrexia

8 Growth and Development, and Body Orientation

In this chapter you will work with terms relating to growth and development of an embryo and other kinds of growing things. You'll cover terms that provide an orientation to the body, something like a road map, to make anatomical descriptions meaningful.

Mini-Glossary

Root Words

cyst	benign	distal
lesion	infiltration	dorsal
polyp	malignant	lateral
papilla	metastasis	medial
papilloma	neoplasm	proximal
papule		ventral

Prefixes

ecto-, exo- (*outer side*)
end-, endo- (*inner, within*)
meso- (*middle*)
circum- (*around*)
peri- (*around about*)
epi- (*over, surrounding*)
sub-, hypo- (*below, under*)
supra-, super- (*above, over*)
infra- (*below, beneath*)

Have you completed the Chapter 7 Review Sheet? We suggest you do it before you begin. It will really help you learn.

Growth and Development

1.
Blastos refers to a germ, seed, sprout, or bud. A *blastoderm* is an aggregation of cells showing the first trace of structure in a microscopic organism. It is the most rudimentary form of a developing embryo and is made up of three primary germ cell layers: the *ectoderm, endoderm,* and *mesoderm.* From these primordial germ layers the embryo develops and becomes a fetus.

2.
Review these definitions and return to them as you need help with the frames that follow.

Ectoderm is the outer layer of cells in the primary germ layers of the developing embryo. It is the origin of:

- the skin (epidermis)
- the mucous membranes of nose, mouth, and anus (epithelium)
- nervous tissue and sensory organs

Mesoderm is the middle of the three primary germ layers of the embryo. It is the origin of:

- all connective tissues
- all body musculature
- blood, cardiovascular, and lymphatic systems
- most of the urogenital system
- the lining of the pericardial, pleural, and peritoneal cavities

Endoderm is the innermost of the three primary germ layers of the embryo, from which are derived:

- the lining of the gut
- its glands (spleen, pancreas, liver)
- component structures of the gut (esophagus, stomach, intestine, colon)
- the respiratory tract

3.
Ectoderm is the outer layer of cells. Endoderm is the innermost of the three germ layers. Mesoderm is the middle layer of three primary germ layers in the developing embryo. Write a meaning for each of the prefixes:

inner, inside	endo- means ________________.
middle	meso- means ________________.
outer, outside	ecto- means ________________.

mesoderm mēz′ ō derm	4. Which primary germ layer originates all connective tissues and all body musculature? ________________
mesoderm	5. The pleura is a watery, mucoid-surfaced membrane enveloping the lungs and lining the walls of the thoracic cavity. From which germ layer does it arise? ________________
ectoderm ek′ tō derm	6. Which of the three embryonic germ layers gives rise to the nervous system and the organs of special sense? ________________
endoderm en′ dō derm	7. The primative gut tract and its associated glands (organs) develop from which germ layer of the embryo? ________________
ectoderm	8. The skin, including mucous membranes exposed to the environment, is derived from the primary germ layer called the ________________.
endoderm ectoderm mesoderm mēz′ ō derm	9. The innermost of the three primary germ layers of the embryo is the ________________. The outside layer of cells in the embryo is the ________________. The middle of the three primary germ layers is the ________________.
of, or pertaining to, outside the cell	10. Now let's try out those new prefixes. Write a meaning for each of the following: ectocytic ________________ ________________

inflammation of inside of the heart	endocarditis ______________________
examination by looking inside of (a body cavity)	endoscopy ______________________
examination of inside the bladder	endocystoscopy ______________________

11.
Gen/o is the combining form to denote originating or production.

Ectogenous means originating outside of a cell or an organism. Underline the part of the term meaning originating or produced.

ecto<u>genous</u> ek toj′ en us	Ectogenous
originating or produced inside of (a cell) en doj′ en us	What does endogenous mean? ______________________

12.
Topos, top/o means place or location. Sometimes a pregnancy begins in the fallopian tube instead of within the uterus. A pregnancy can also implant in the gut, abdomen, cervix, or lining of the uterus. These atypical placement pregnancies are called ectopic pregnancies.

pregnancy outside of its normal location	What is an ectopic pregnancy? ______________________

13.

ectopic ek top′ ik	A pregnancy beginning in the abdominal cavity instead of the womb is called an ______________ pregnancy.

14.
Let's review before going on. From the suggested answers, select the best term for each brief definition.

SUGGESTED ANSWERS:

ecto-, exo-	endo-, en-, end-
ectopic	endocranial
ectocytic	endogenous
meso-	mesoderm

ecto- (exo-)	outside (prefix) ______________________
meso-	middle (prefix) ______________________

endo- (en- or end-)	inside (prefix) ____
mesoderm	middle germ cell layer ____
endogenous	originating inside ____
ectocytic	pertaining to outside the cell ____
ectopic	out of its normal place ____
endocranial	pertaining to inside the head ____

Growths and Other Abnormal Tissues

15.
In this section you'll work with more terms relating to growth. Growing means to increase progressively in size. However, growth may be normal and purposeful, or abnormal and useless. Here are some terms used to describe abnormal growth.

neoplasm
nē′ ō plazm

16.
Neo- means new; *-plasm* means thing formed. Neoplasm is a new formation of tissue. It is abnormal because it serves no useful function and grows at the expense of a healthy body. Any tissue growing autonomously and that has no useful function is a ____.

neoplasm

17.
A tumor is a swelling or enlargement. It is an autonomous new growth of tissue. It is a mass of tissue without a function. Another word for tumor is ____.

growth of tissue that serves no useful purpose

18.
Neoplasm and tumor are interchangeable terms. They both mean an autonomous new ____
____.

tissue
examines

19.
Bio- means life; *-opsy* means appearance, sight. A biopsy is removing tissue from a living body and examining it under a microscope.

To make a diagnosis, a physician usually biopsies a tumor or neoplasm. This means the physician removes a piece of living ____ and ____ it under a microscope.

20.
A neoplasm (tumor) growing in or on the human body can be classified as either malignant or benign.

Malignant means it's of a bad kind, growing worse, resisting treatment, and tending or threatening to produce death.

benign
bē nīn′
malignant
ma lig′ nant

Benign means it's mild, not spreading, not recurrent, and not malignant. Tumors may be of uncertain behavior, but usually are classified either as ________________ or ________________.

21.
To determine what kind of neoplasm a patient has, the physician removes a piece of the living tumor tissue and examines it under a microscope. What is this procedure called? ________________

biopsy

22.
A biopsy report indicates a patient's abnormal growth is of a bad kind. It will grow worse, resist treatment, and tend to be life-threatening. The diagnosis is ________________ neoplasm.
(malignant/benign)

malignant

23.
A nonmalignant neoplasm is an abnormal tissue mass that does not spread, and is not likely to recur. The growth is ________________.
(malignant/benign)

benign

24.
A procedure that determines whether a neoplasm is benign or malignant is a ________________.

biopsy

25.
A benign neoplasm is mild, does not spread or recur, and is not ________________.
(the other kind)

malignant

26.
Infiltration means slipping into and between normal cells of the body.

Malignant tumor cells may spread by slipping into and between normal body cells. Malignant cells multiply rapidly and take up nourishment and space, crowding out the normal cells. This method of spreading is called direct extension or ________________.

infiltration

27.
Metastasis means movement of cells (especially cancer cells) from one part of the body to another.

Meta- means after, beyond, among, over; *-stasis* means a standing, a location, or a place.

metastasis me tas′ tə sis	Malignant tumor cells migrate to another location and take up a standing in another organ or part of the body. This method of spreading the disease is called invasion by ________.
	28.
location	Metastasis is the movement of malignant tumor cells from the primary location over to another ________.
	29.
infiltration or direct extension metastasis	There are two methods by which a malignant neoplasm spreads, grows larger, and becomes more threatening. Malignant cells may slip into and between normal cells. This is called ________ ________. Or tumor cells may move beyond the primary site and take up a standing in another location of the body. This spreading method is called ________.
	30.
infiltration metastasis	Unlike malignant neoplasms, benign growths do not spread by ________ or ________.
	31.
	Here's a quick review. Select a term from the suggested answers that best fits each brief definition. Write your selection in the space provided.
	malignant — neoplasm/tumor tumor/neoplasm — biopsy benign — infiltration metastasize
biopsy	remove tissue for examination ________
benign	mild, not malignant ________
neoplasm/tumor	new, abnormal tissue mass ________
tumor/neoplasm	tissue mass, no useful purpose ________
malignant	abnormal growth that threatens death ________
infiltration	slipping into and between normal cells ________
metastasize (me tās′ tə sīz)	cells relocate to new location, organ ________
	32.
	There are many other terms that mean abnormal conditions, changes, or growths. Here are a few of the more common ones.

33.
Lesion is an area of unhealthy (morbid) tissue, such as an injury, wound, burn, or infected patch of skin.

lesion
lē′ zhun

Any morbid change in the structure of an organ or a body part due to injury or disease is called a ________________.

34.
An infected finger is a lesion because there has been a morbid change in the finger tissues. What does morbid mean?

diseased, unhealthy

____

35.
In Alzheimer's disease there are morbid changes in brain tissue. These unhealthy changes in brain structure are also called ______________.

lesions

36.
An injury, a burn, and an infected finger are examples of lesions because the part of the body involved has undergone a __________ (unhealthy) change.

morbid

37.
A lesion is any morbid change in the structure of an organ or part due to injury or disease. Check each item that is *not* a lesion.

☒ chicken pox is a disease; the pox are lesions

- ☐ duodenal ulcer
- ☐ skinned knees
- ☐ scalding burn of the hand
- ☐ abrasion of the elbow
- ☐ chicken pox
- ☐ infected toenail

38.
Poison ivy leaves may irritate the skin and cause blisters. These unhealthy changes in the structure of the skin are called ____________.

lesions

39.
Build a word meaning a hurt, an injury, or any unhealthy area of any organ or part: ________________.

lesion

40.
What does morbid mean? ______________________________

unhealthy, diseased

41.
In earlier units you learned that cyst means bladder.

inflammation of the bladder — Cystitis means ______________________.

examination of the inside of the bladder — Endocystoscopy means ______________________.

excision (or removal) of the gallbladder — Cholecystectomy means ______________________.

42.
Cyst also means a closed sac or pouch that contains fluid, semifluid, or solid material.

sac or pouch — A cyst is a closed ______________.

fluid, semifluid, or solid material — It contains ______________________.

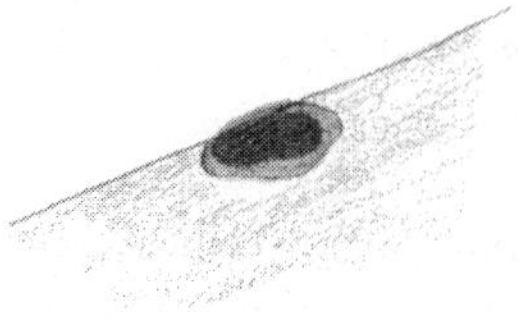

Figure 8.1 Cyst

43.
cyst — A malfunctioning ovary may develop a closed sac or pouch containing fluid. This is called an ovarian ______________.

44.
a cyst containing fluid (water) — What is a hydrocyst? ______________________

a sac that contains fluid or even solid material — Cyst means ______________________.

45.
A physician doesn't usually drain a cyst of its contents because it would only fill again. Instead, a surgeon completely excises the cyst.

cystectomy — Write a term meaning surgical removal of a cyst: ______________.

46.
Polyp is a tumor with a little foot, or stem. A polyp is usually a benign tumor. That means it is not ________________________,
(the other kind)

pol′ ip
malignant

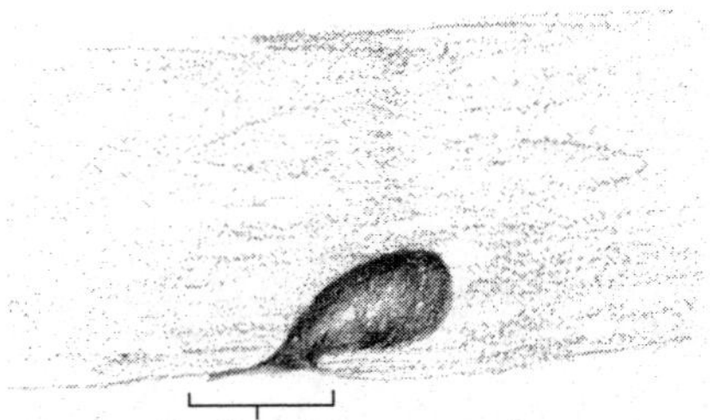

Figure 8.2 Polyp

it grows ________________________, and it does *not* spread by
(fast/slowly)

________________________ or ________________________.

slowly
infiltration
metastasis

47.
A polyp is a specific type of tumor or neoplasm. It's an abnormal, useless new growth that stands on a stem or a little ________________.

foot

48.
Vascular organs such as the nose, uterus, and rectum commonly develop polyps. Polyps bleed easily and usually are removed surgically. Build a word for excision of polyps: ________________________.

polypectomy

What does vascular mean? This is a good time to use a dictionary.

____

49.
A lesion is an area of ________________________ tissue.

unhealthy

Give some examples of lesions: ____
____.

burn, injury, infection

50.
Cyst has two different meanings.

Cyst means ________________________.
a part of the body

bladder

Cyst also means ____.
definition

a sac containing fluid or semifluid

51.

tumor/neoplasm
little foot, or stem

A polyp is a specific kind of ________________.
A polyp has a ________________.

52.
Papilla is a small nipplelike protuberance or elevation. It may be located anywhere on the body, and may be normal or abnormal.

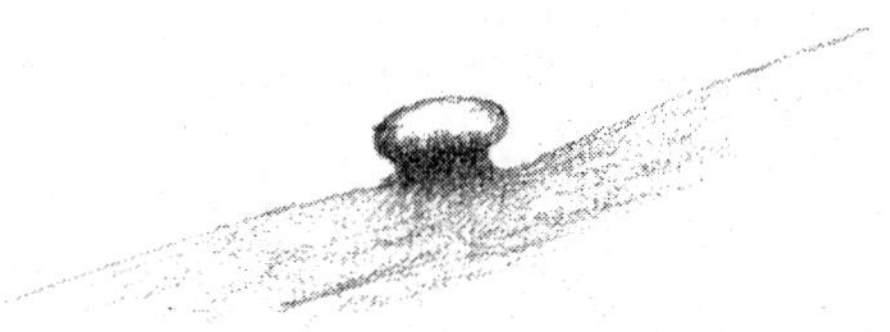

Figure 8.3 Papilla

small, nipplelike structures

Taste buds are small nipplelike structures on the surface of the tongue. They account for the four fundamental taste sensations: sweet, bitter, sour, and salt. Stand in front of a mirror; stick your tongue way out. You will see papillae (plural) on the back of your tongue. Describe them: ________________.

53.

papilla
pa pil′ ə

The nipple of the mammary gland (breast) is called a mammary ________________.

54.

pap i lō′ mä

Papilloma is a hypertrophied papilla covered by a layer of skin. What is the shape of a papilloma?

nipplelike

____

55.

pap′ yo͞ol

Papule is a pimple. It's a red elevated spot on the skin. It's solid and circumscribed. Papular lesions appear on the skin in smallpox, measles, and chicken pox.

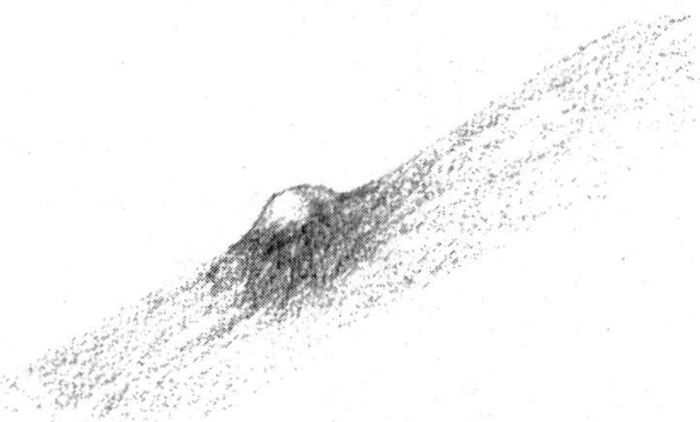

Figure 8.4 Papule

spots — They are elevated red ________________ on the skin.

circumscribed — They are solid and ________________.

56.
Excrescence: ex means out; *crescence* means to grow. Excrescence is a useless structure growing out of the surface of a part such as a wart or mole.

The Wicked Witch of the West had a big wart growing on the tip of her nose. A medical term for this disfiguring outgrowth is ________________.

excrescence
eks kres′ ens

Figure 8.5 Excrescence

57.
Condyloma is a wartlike growth of the skin, occurring in the genital area. The main difference between an excrescence and a condyloma is where the lesion is located. An excrescence may appear anywhere on the surface of the body (even on the end of your nose).
But a wartlike skin growth in the genital area is called a ________________.

kon di lō′ mä
condyloma

58.
An excrescence, a papilloma, a condyloma, and a papule are all lesions of the skin. That means the area of the skin involved is considered ________________.

morbid, unhealthy

59.
Papillae (plural) may be normal structures on the body that have important functions. A taste bud is a papilla. Describe what it looks like: ________________.

pa pil′ ē (pl.)
small, nipplelike protuberance

(For help in learning the plural forms, see Appendix B: Forming Plurals.)

60.
Label each of the following illustrations.

a. papule
b. polyp
c. cyst
d. papilloma

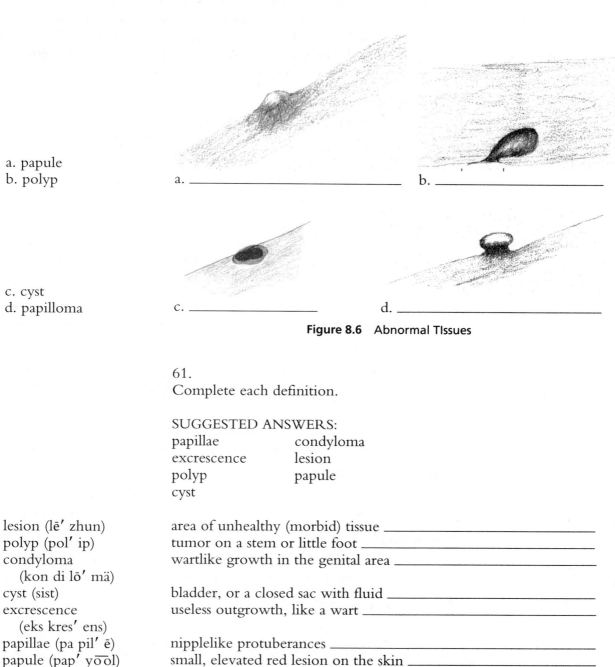

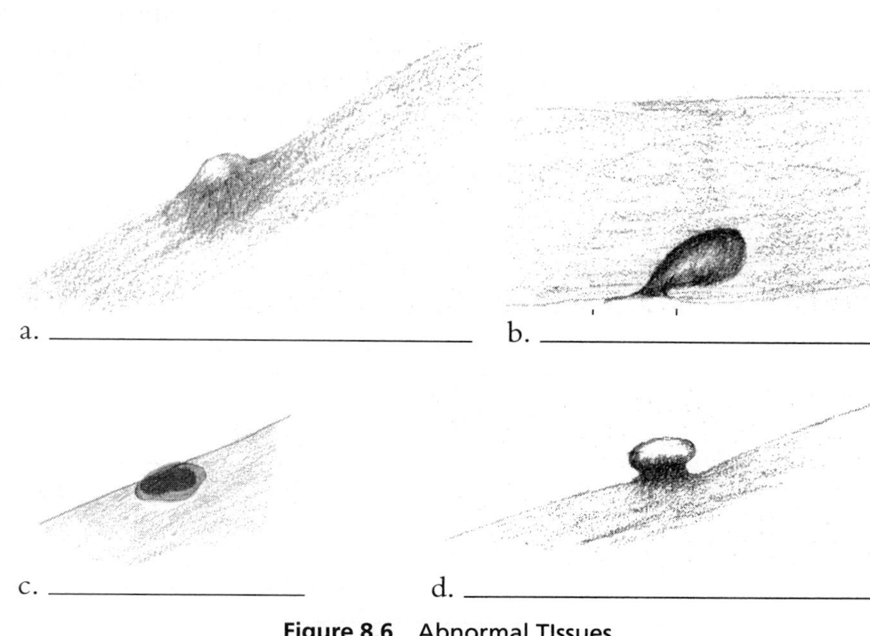

Figure 8.6 Abnormal TIssues

61.
Complete each definition.

SUGGESTED ANSWERS:

papillae	condyloma
excrescence	lesion
polyp	papule
cyst	

lesion (lē′ zhun)	area of unhealthy (morbid) tissue ______
polyp (pol′ ip)	tumor on a stem or little foot ______
condyloma (kon di lō′ mä)	wartlike growth in the genital area ______
cyst (sist)	bladder, or a closed sac with fluid ______
excrescence (eks kres′ ens)	useless outgrowth, like a wart ______
papillae (pa pil′ ē)	nipplelike protuberances ______
papule (pap′ yo͞ol)	small, elevated red lesion on the skin ______

62.

Here's an independent learning exercise for you. These are words related to treatments and consequences of malignant neoplasms. Look up each one in your medical dictionary. Explore it thoroughly; pronounce it several times. Then write a brief definition for each. Do this exercise even if you think you know what the terms mean. Sometimes you'll be surprised!

abdominal paracentesis

____

____

alopecia

____

____

anastomosis

____

____

cauterization

____

____

chemotherapy

____

____

dehiscence

____

____

necrobiosis

____

____

radiation

____

____

radical resection

____

____

Orientation

63.
Neoplasms, cysts, and lesions occur anywhere on the surface of the body and inside, under, and around organs and structures. Health care providers use specific terms to describe where lesions and other morbid conditions are located relative to parts of the body. This assists other providers in following a condition through treatment.

64.
Ventral means on or near the belly, or the side of the body where the belly is located.

back

Dorsal is the opposite of ventral; it means on or near the ________.

Label the illustrations.

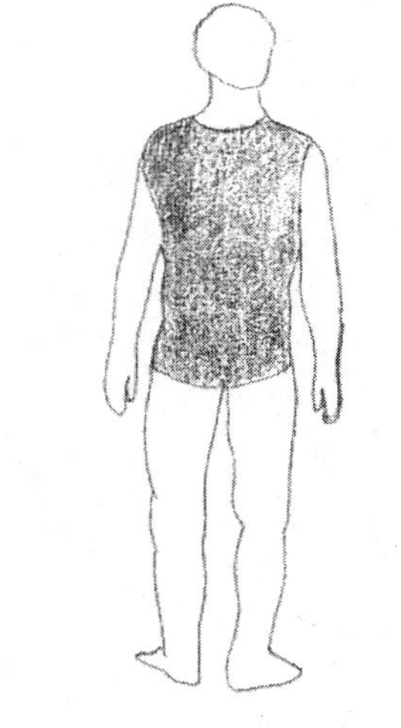

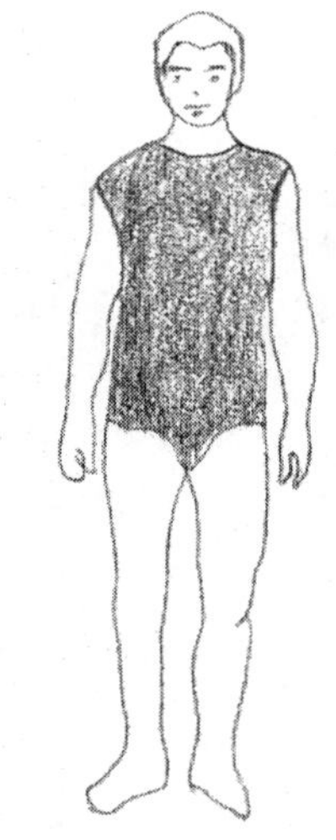

a. dorsal
b. ven′ tral
ven′ tral

a. ________ b. ________

Figure 8.7

65.

belly
back

Ventral, ventr/o means on or near the ________.
Dorsal, dors/o means on or near the ________.

66.
Try these.

backache — Dorsalgia means ______________________.

incision into the belly — Ventrotomy means ______________________.

67.
of or pertaining to belly to back — What do you think ventrodorsad means? ______________________

A bullet penetrated the abdominal wall, traveled through the belly, and exited through the back. The bullet's path may be described as ______________________.

ventrodorsad
ven trō dor′ säd

68.
The *midline,* or median, is an imaginary line dividing the body into right and left halves.

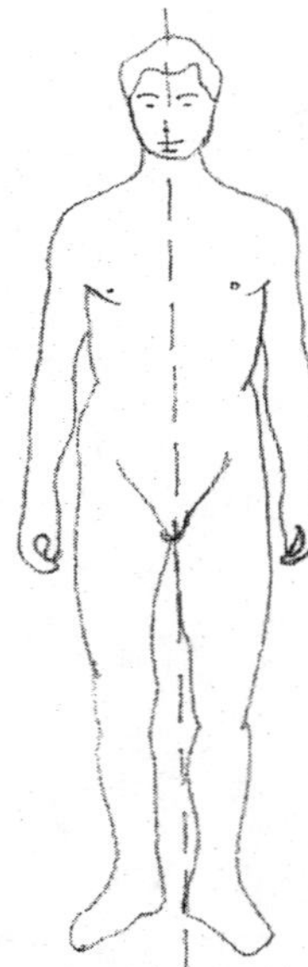

Figure 8.8 Midline of the Body

Lateral means farther from the midline.

Medial means closer to the midline.

closer — Medial means ______________________ to the midline.

Which is nearer the midline, your shoulder or your nipple?

nipple — ______________________

	69.
lateral	Which corner of your eye is nearest your ear? ________ (medial/lateral)
medial	Which side of your knee knocks the other knee? ________ (medial/lateral)
	70.
farther	Lateral means ________ from the midline.
closer	Medial means ________ to the midline.
on the midline	Where is your umbilicus located? ________
	71.
	Let's describe a relative position in another way. *Distal* means remote, or farthest, from the point of attachment to the trunk.
nearest	*Proximal* means the opposite. Proximal means ________ (farthest/nearest) to the point of attachment to the trunk.
	72.
hand	Which is distal, your elbow or your hand? ________
proximal	On which end of your finger do you wear a ring? ________ (distal/proximal)
	73.
distal	Your forearm bone has two ends. Your hand is attached to the ________ (distal/proximal) end.
proximal	Your upper arm is located on the ________ (distal/proximal) end.
	74.
proximal	A part of the body located nearest its attachment to the trunk is described as ________.
distal	A part located farthest from its attachment to the trunk is described as ________.
	75.
farthest from the attachment to the trunk	The fingers are distal to all other parts of the arm. What does distal mean? ________ ________

	76.
nearest to the attachment to the trunk	Describe the location of a part that is proximal: ______________________________ ____________.
	77.
	Here's a review of what you just covered. Select the best term from the suggested answers to complete each definition.
	SUGGESTED ANSWERS: distal proximal medial lateral ventral midline dorsal
dorsal	near or on the back ______________________
ventral	near or on the belly ______________________
midline	divides body into right and left halves ______________
lateral	farther from the midline ______________________
medial	nearer to the midline ______________________
distal	farthest from the attachment to the trunk ____________
proximal	nearest to the attachment to the trunk ____________
	78.
	Here are some prefixes indicating place or relative position:
	Peri-, circum- means around, about, surrounding,
	Write a meaning for each of the following:
pertaining to around the tonsil	Peri/tonsillar ______________________ ______________
relating to around the belly button	Peri/umbilical ______________________ ______________
	79.
diseased (unhealthy) tissue around the teeth	What is peri/dent/al (peri/dont/al) gum disease? ____________ ______________________ ____________
around	Peri- means ______________.

80.

Circum- is another prefix meaning ________. *Duct/ion* means moving.

around

Ab/duct/ion is moving away. Circum/duction means ________ ________.

moving around

81.

A wheal (hives) is a round patch of unhealthy skin with a ring of normal tissue at its circumference. A wheal appears as a round red spot. We usually say a wheal is ________-scribed.

circum(-scribed)

82.

A boil also has an outer limit where the circumference of the lesion becomes normal. Because it appears to have a border around its circumference, you may also describe a boil as a ________ lesion.

circumscribed

83.

Perioral and circumoral have the same meaning. Write the meaning: ________.

relating to around the mouth

Write a meaning for circumrenal, perirenal: ________ ________.

pertaining to around or surrounding the kidney

84.

Look over the following terms and their meanings and then complete the frames that follow. Come back to this frame whenever you need help.

epi-	upon, over (surrounding or covering)
extra-	without, outside of
infra-	below, beneath, under
sub-, hypo-	below, beneath, less than normal
supra-, super-	above, superior, in the upper part of

85.

The epi/gastric region is the region of the belly over or upon the stomach. Refer to Figure 8.9 on page 189.

Epi/gastralgia means ________ ________ ________.

pain in the area of the belly over the stomach

hernia in the area of the belly over the stomach

Epi/gastrocele means ____
______________________________.

86.
Epi/cranium refers to the tissues (muscle and skin) that cover and surround the cranium. What do you think epi/dermis means? ______

the skin (that covers the entire body)

____.

87.
Go back to the definitions in Frame 84. The prefix extra- means

without, outside of

____.

outside the uterus

Extra/uterine means ______________________________.

outside the edges or outer limits of a structure or organ

Extra/marginal means ____
______________________________.

88.
Again use the definitions to help you. The prefix *infra*- means

below, beneath, under

____.

pertaining to an area under, below the kneecap

Patella means kneecap. What does infra/patellar mean? ___________
____.

beneath, under the kneecap

Sub/patellar means ____
______________________________.

89.
Infra- and sub- usually are interchangeable terms. Complete the alternate terms and write a meaning:

infra (-mammary)

______________________-mammary

sub (-mammary)

______________________-mammary

below the breast

meaning ______________________________.

90.
Sub- and hypo- are often interchangeable also.

under the tongue

Sub/lingual means ______________________________.

under the tongue

Hypo/glossal means ______________________________.

below, beneath, less than normal infra- hypo-	91. The prefix sub- means ____. What other two prefixes often are interchangeable and mean the same thing as sub- ? ________________ and ________________
pertaining to below the breastbone	92. Sternum is the breastbone. Write a meaning for sub/sternal: ____.
infrasternal	Use another prefix and build another term that means the same thing: ____________________.
suprasternal	93. Build a term that means pertaining to above the sternum: ____________________.

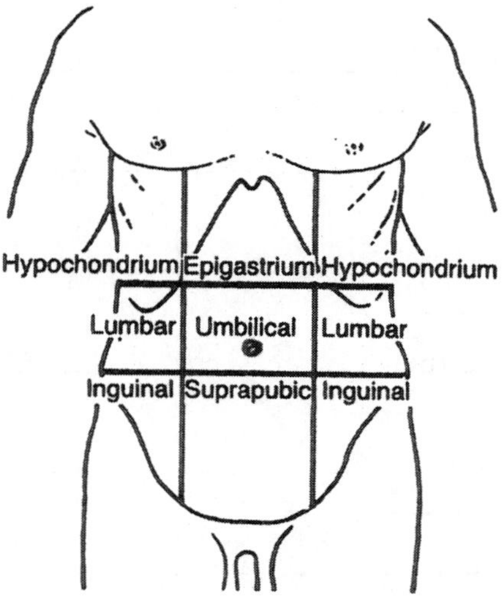

Figure 8.9 Regions of the Abdomen

	94. Refer to Figure 8.9 to help you complete the next few frames.
suprapubic	95. Sub/pubic refers to an area beneath the pubic arch (bone). Build a term meaning relating to the area above the pubic arch: ____________________.
umbilicus or belly button	Umbilical is the term meaning relating to the area that is near/around the ____.

beneath the ribs (these floating ribs are composed mostly of cartilage)

96.
Chondros means cartilage (of ribs). Literally, hypochondrium means the area ____________________.

inguinal
ing′ gwi nal

97.
Look at Figure 8.9, Regions of the Abdomen. Lumbar relates to the loin. It is the part of the back and sides between the ribs and the pelvis. What area is below the lumbar region? ____________

When describing regions of the abdomen that occur on both sides, you may say left or right to discriminate. Use the client as a point of reference, that is, the client's left side lumbar region is called left lumbar.

98.
Write a meaning for each of the following terms.

pertaining to around the umbilicus

peri/umbilical ____________________

relating to below the abdomen

sub/abdominal ____________________

relating to above the loin

supra/lumbar ____________________

pertaining to below the pubic arch

infra/pubic ____________________

pertaining to around the intestine

circum/intestinal ____________________

pertaining to under the skin

hypo/dermic ____________________

relating to outside the field of vision

extra/visual ____________________

pertaining to over the stomach

epigastric ____________________

99.
In this chapter you worked with 36 new medical terms. Practice pronouncing them. Then take the Chapter 8 Self-Test.

benign (bē nīn′)	circumocular
biopsy	circumscribed

condyloma (kon di lō′ mä)
cyst (sist)
distal
dorsal
ectoderm (ek tō derm)
ectopic (ek top′ ik)
endocystoscopy (en dō sis tos′ ko pē)
endogenous (en doj′ ə nus)
epigastric (ep ē gas′ trik)
excrescence (eks kres′ ens)
extrasensory (eks tra sen′ sō rē)
hypodermic (hī pō derm′ ik)
infiltration
inframammary (in fra mam′ ə rē)
lateral
lesion
lumbar
malignant (ma lig′ nant)
medial
mesoderm (mēz′ ō derm)
metastasis (me tas′ ta sis)
neoplasm (nē ō plazm)
papilla (pa pil′ ə)
papilloma (pap i lō′ mä)
papules (pap′ yo͞ols)
periumbilical (per′ ē um bil′ i k'l)
polyp (pol′ ip)
proximal (prox′ si mal)
subpatellar (sub pa tel′ ar)
suprapubic (su pra pyo͞o′ bik)
tumor
ventral

Chapter 8 Self-Test

Part 1

From the right, select the correct meaning for each of the following often-used medical terms.

_____ 1. Endocystoscopy
_____ 2. Lesion
_____ 3. Circumocular
_____ 4. Distal
_____ 5. Endocranial
_____ 6. Epigastric
_____ 7. Biopsy
_____ 8. Neoplasm
_____ 9. Ectoderm
_____ 10. Metastasis
_____ 11. Malignant
_____ 12. Benign
_____ 13. Infiltration
_____ 14. Proximal
_____ 15. Ectopic

a. Farthest point from trunk attachment
b. Outside layer of germ cells
c. Not spreading, not malignant
d. Pertaining to inside the head vault
e. Pertaining to around the eye
f. Slipping into and between normal cells
g. Pertaining to the area over the stomach
h. Cells spread to new location, organ
i. Removal of tissue for examination
j. New, abnormal tissue formation
k. Morbid tissue
l. Nearest the attachment to the trunk
m. A bad kind, tending to threaten death
n. Occurring outside the normal place
o. Examination inside the bladder

Part 2

Write the medical term for each of the following brief definitions.

1. Nipple-like protuberance ________________
2. New, abnormal tissue without a purpose ________________
3. Useless structure growing out of the skin (wart) ________________
4. Spread of malignant cells to new location, organ ________________
5. Pertaining to on or near the back ________________
6. Farthest point from trunk attachment ________________
7. Closed sac or pouch containing fluid ________________
8. Removal of tissue for examination ________________
9. Wartlike growth in the genital area Con________________
10. Slipping into and between normal cells ________________
11. Not spreading, not malignant ________________
12. Below the mammary gland ________________
13. Tumor with a little foot ________________
14. Nearest point of trunk attachment ________________
15. Unhealthy, diseased area of tissue ________________

ANSWERS

Part 1	*Part 2*
1. o	1. Papilla
2. k	2. Neoplasm/tumor
3. e	3. Excrescence
4. a	4. Metastasis
5. d	5. Dorsal
6. g	6. Distal
7. i	7. Cyst
8. j	8. Biopsy
9. b	9. Condyloma

10. h	10. Infiltration
11. m	11. Benign
12. c	12. Inframammary
13. f	13. Polyp
14. l	14. Proximal
15. n	15. Lesion

9 Gynecology, Pregnancy, and Childbirth

This chapter covers medical terms used in gynecology, pregnancy, and childbirth. This lesson may be difficult at times, so be kind to yourself and go slowly. If you don't get the right answers the first time you work through a sequence, try again before moving on. Here are the whole terms, word roots, prefixes, and suffixes you'll work with.

Mini-Glossary

Root Words

amni/o, amniot/o (*fetal sac*)
gravid/a (*with child*)
gyn/o, gynec/o (*woman*)
hyster/o (*uterus*)
mamm/o (*breast*)
mast/o (*breast*)
men/o (*menses, menstruation*)
metr/o (*uterus*)
para (*bear, bring forth*)

Prefixes

multi- (*many*)
nulli- (*none*)
oligo- (*little, small, scanty*)
post- (*after*)
pre- (*before*)
primi- (*first*)
secundi- (*second*)

Suffixes

-ary (*of or pertaining to*)
-atrophy (*undernourished, wasting*)
-dynia (*pain, painful*)
-mania (*madness*)
-pathy (*disease*)
-phobia (*excessive fear*)

Important Words

climacteric
conception
embryo
episiotomy
fetus
gestation

involution
labor
menopause
ovum
parturition
perineum
peritoneum
placenta
pudenda
puerperium

Do yourself a big favor. Complete the Review Sheet for Chapter 8 before you tackle this unit.

Terms of Gynecology

1.
Gyn, gynec/o means woman. Gynecology is the study of the female reproductive organs and breasts. Simply put, it is the field of medicine dealing with diseases of whom? ____________________

women

Before continuing, go to Figure 4.2, The Female Reproductive Organs. Review the illustration and read again the description that follows.

2.
Gyn/o/pathic means pertaining to diseases of female reproductive organs. What do you think gyn/o/plasty means? ____________________

gī′ nō plas tē or jin′ ō plas tē
plastic surgery of female reproductive organs

3.
Mania means madness. *Phobia* means excessive fear. Gynecomania is an abnormal sex drive and desire in the male of the species. What do you think gyne/phobia means? ____________________

gī ne fo′ bē a
fear of women

4.
The physician who specializes in female disorders is called a ____________________.

gynecologist
gī ne kol′ ō jist

5.
Human beings are mammals. Mammals have glands that secrete milk for nourishing their offspring. In plain English, mammary gland refers to ____________________.

breast

6.
These next two terms often are interchangeable. However, we use one term more often than the other. In this lesson you'll be using the *preferred terms*. Let's see what this means:

breast	*Mamm, mamm/o* refers to mammary gland, or breast; *mast, mast/o* also refers to ________________.
mam ī′ tis, mast ī′ tis inflammation of the mammary gland (breast) preferred	7. Mamm/itis and mast/itis both mean ____ ________________________________. Mastitis is the term used most often, so we say it is the ________________ term.
ma mog′ ra fē mamm/o/graphy X ray exam of the breast	8. Break down each of the following preferred terms and write its meaning. Mammography, ____________ / _____ / ______________, means ____ ___________.
mas tek′ tō mē mast/ectomy surgical removal of a breast	Mastectomy, ____________ / ______________, means ____ ___________.
mastotomy mas tot′ ō mē incision into the breast mastitis inflammation of the breast mastopathy mas top′ a thē disease of the mammary gland	9. Using the word root or combining form, mast, mast/o, add a suffix from the list and build a preferred term. Write its meaning in the space provided. -otomy -itis -pathy m ________________ means ____ ______________ m ________________ means ____ ______________ m ________________ means ____ ______________
mastoptosis mas top tō′ sis	10. Very large breasts that hang down, or droop, are described as pendulous. The suffix for hanging or drooping is -ptosis. Construct a word meaning pendulous breast: ________________.

11.
Here's an interesting term that doesn't follow the rules. Let's look at the parts. Gynec/o means woman; mastia means breast.

gī ne kō mas′ tē a
woman's breast

Gynecomastia literally means ______________________.

In actual use it means abnormally large mammary glands in the male; sometimes they secrete milk.

12.
This time use mamm, mamm/o. Build a term with each of the following suffixes and write its meaning:

-gram -ary

mam′ ō gram
mammogram
X ray picture of the breast

m ______________
means ______________________________

mam′ a rē
mammary
pertaining to the mammary gland

m ______________
means ______________________________

13.
Mamm/o/pexy means surgical correction (fixation) of large hanging breasts. What does mamm/o/plasty mean? ______________

mam′ ō plas tē
plastic surgery of the mammary gland

14.
Mast/aden/itis means inflammation of the mammary gland. Write a meaning for each of the following:

mast′ ad nī tis
mast′ ad nō′ ma
tumor of the mammary gland

mastadenoma ______________________________

mas tō kar cin ō′ ma
cancerous tumor of the mammary gland

mastocarcinoma ______________________________

15.
The study or science dealing with the physical, chemical, and biologic properties of neoplasms including causation, pathogenesis, and treatment is oncology. What does mastoncus mean? ______________

mas tong′ kus
(any) tumor of the breast

mast/algia
mast al′ jē ə

16.
Mast/o/dynia means painful breast. Using another suffix you know, build another word that also means pain in the breast:
mast/____________________.

17.
Here's a quick review. Select a term from the suggested answers that best fits each brief definition. Write your selection in the space provided.

mastectomy	mastopathy
mastoptosis	gynecomastia
mastoncus	mastopexy

Answer	Definition
mastopathy mas top′ a thē	disease of the mammary glands ____________________
gynecomastia	women's breasts (on a man) ____________________
mastectomy	surgical removal of the breast ____________________
mastoptosis	pendulous breasts ____________________
mastoncus	any tumor of the breast ____________________
mastopexy mas′ tō pex′ sē	surgical fixation of pendulous breasts ____________________

18.
Now try these.

mammoplasty	mammary
mammology	mammalgia (mastodynia)
mammography	gynecophobia

Answer	Definition
mammography	X ray study of the breast ____________________
mammalgia (mastodynia)	painful breast ____
mammology	science and study of the breast ____________________
gynecophobia	fear of women ____________________
mammary	pertaining to the breast ____________________
mammoplasty	surgical reconstruction of the breast ____________________

19.
Mamma mē′ a, you're doing very well!

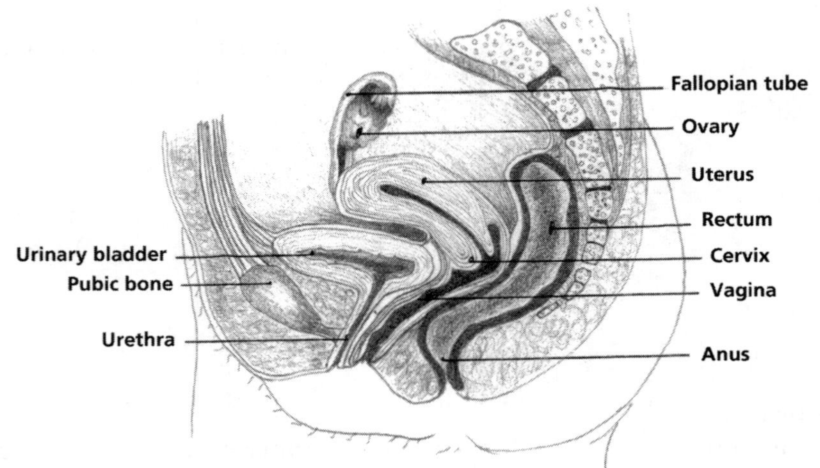

Figure 9.1 The Female Reproductive Organs (Midline Section)

See pages 75–76 for a description of the female reproductive organs.

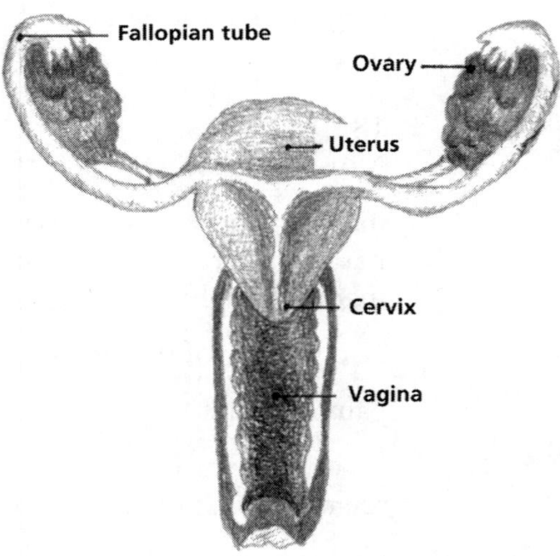

Figure 9.2 The Female Reproductive Organs (Anterior View)

ovary (oophor/o)
fallopian tube (salping/o)
uterus (hyster/o, metr/o)
uterine cervix (cerv/i)
vagina (vagin/o)
breast (mamm/o, mast/o)
menses (men/o)
muscle (my/o)
bladder (cyst/o)
urethra (urethr/o)

20.
Here are two more terms with nearly identical meanings. Refer to Figures 9.1 and 9.2.

Hyster, hyster/o means uterus. *Metr, metr/o* also means ________________.

uterus

21.
Hyster/o usually refers to the uterus as a whole organ. Metr/o usually refers to the tissues of the ________________.

uterus

22.
There are exceptions to the rule, but in general hyster/o means the uterus as a ________________ organ. Metr/o refers to the ________________ of the organ.

whole
tissues

23.
Metr/itis means an inflammation of the uterine tissues (linings, muscles, etc.). Metr/o/paralysis means paralysis of ________________ ________________.

(muscle) tissues of the uterus

24.
Hyster/o/tomy means incision into the uterus (perhaps to remove a solid tumor). My-, myo- means muscle. What does hyster/o/my/oma mean? ________________ ________________

muscle tumor of the uterus

25.
Using the word roots hyster, hyster/o, add a suffix from the list and build a new word. Write its meaning in the space provided:

-ectomy -pathy

h ________________
means ________________ ________________

hysterectomy
his ter rek′ tō mē
surgical removal of the uterus

h ________________
means ________________ ________________

hysteropathy
his ter op′ ō thē
disease of the uterus

26.
Try it again using metr or metr/o. Build a term and then write its meaning:

-scope -itis
-atrophy (wasting away, diminishing in size)

metroscope mēt′ rō skōp instrument for examining the uterus	m ______________________ means ____________________________________ __________________
metritis mē trī′ tis inflammation of uterine tissues	m ______________________ means ____________________________________ __________________
metratrophy mē tra′ trō fē uterine tissue atrophy	m ______________________ means ____________________________________ __________________

27.
Use the word roots metr/, metr/o with the following suffixes to make a new word that fits each of the definitions:

-orrhagia means hemorrhage
-orrhea means flow or discharge

metrorrhagia mē trō rā′ jē ə	uterine hemorrhage __________________;
metrorrhea mē trō rē′ ə	discharge from the uterus (mucus or pus) __________________.

28.
Here are two suffixes that can be confusing:

-orrhexis means rupture (bursting open);
-ocele means hernia or rupture.

The difference between them is the degree of severity of the outcome; the first has a high mortality.

Build a term meaning ruptured uterus (ruptured during labor threatening the mother's life and perhaps the infant's):

hysterorrhexis his′ ter ō rek′ sis	hyster__________________.

Build a term meaning uterine hernia (to be repaired by a surgeon):

hysterocele his′ ter ō sēl	hyster__________________.

29.
Endo/metr/ium refers to the inside lining of the uterus. Myo/metr/ium refers to the muscle layer of the uterus.

Build a term meaning inflammation of the inside lining and muscle layers of the uterus:

endo/myo/metr/itis
en dō mī ō mē trī′ tis

____________ / ____________ / ____________ / ____________.
inside muscle uterus inflammation

30.
Two word roots and their combining forms refer to the uterus. They are ____________ and ____________.

hyster, hyster/o
metr, metr/o

31.
The term meaning the whole organ is ____________. The term referring to the tissues of the organ is ____________.

hyster/o
metr/o

32.
Now let's look at a uterine function. *Menses, men/o* means monthly flow of bloody fluid from the uterus. Menstruation is the function of discharging the menses. Men/o in any word should make you think of ____________.

menstruation
men strū ā′ shun

33.
Men/orrhea means free flow of menses, also known as menstruation. Dys/men/orrhea means ____________.

dis men ō rē′ a
difficult or painful menstruation

34.
Men/orrh/algia also means ____________
____________.

me nor al′ jē a
painful flow of menses

35.
Try this.

Men/o/metr/orrhagia means ____________
____
____________.

men ō mē trō rā′ jē ə
excessive bleeding (hemorrhage) from the uterus during menstruation

36.
Menopause is a normal physiological condition of a mature woman. It's an event that ends a woman's menstrual life. This event marks the end of her childbearing period. It means the permanent cessation of ____________.

menses
men′ sēs

37.
Menopause means the permanent cessation of the menses. It marks the end of a woman's capability for bearing ________________.

children

38.
Climacteric is a *transitional period* of life sometimes called the change of life. It is a period between ages 45 and 60 when many changes take place in a woman's body. At the end of this transitional period, she no longer experiences menstruation and is no longer capable of bearing a child. The outcome of this transitional period is called ________________________________ ____________.

cessation of menses, or menopause

Climacteric is also called peri__________, or prior to menopause.

menopause

39.
During the female climacteric a key physical change takes place. The ovaries permanently and irreversibly atrophy, ending the reproductive period.

This *transitional period* of life is called the climacteric. The outcome of this transition period is the __________, which means ____________ ____________________.

complete cessation of menses
menopause

40.
The *critical period* of life marking the beginning of the end of childbearing and ending with the onset of menopause is called the ____________________.

climacteric
klī mak′ ter ik

41.
Men also experience a decline in sexual activity in their presenile years. This *change of life period* in a man is called the male ____________________.

climacteric

42.
Menopause ends the body's reproductive function. What word describes the transitional period of critical changes that ends in menopause? ____________________

the climacteric

43.
It's time to review the word combinations you've learned in this section. From the suggested answers, select a term to go with each definition. Write your selection in the space provided.

hysteropathy	mammography
mastodynia	gynecomastia
metrorrhagia	endometritis

Answer	Definition
gynecomastia	woman's breast (in a male) ______
hysteropathy	uterine disease ______
mastodynia	painful breast ______
endometritis	inflammation inside the uterus ______
mammography	X ray examination of the breast ______
metrorrhagia	uterine hemorrhage ______

44.
Here are a few more.

SUGGESTED ANSWERS:

hysterorrhexis	menorrhalgia
amenorrhea	climactric (female)
menopause	metratrophy

Answer	Definition
menopause	permanent cessation of menses ______
amenorrhea	lack of menstruation (temporary) ______
hysterorrhexis	rupture of uterus (during labor) ______
climacteric (female)	change of life transition period ______
menorrhalgia	painful menstruation ______
metratrophy	wasting (diminishing in size) of the uterus ______

Pregnancy and Childbirth

In this section you'll learn one term at a time. First you'll read a brief paragraph defining the new term. Then you'll answer questions and complete statements about it showing you understand what it means. Feel free to refer back to the paragraph as you work through the frames that follow.

Conception means fertilization. It's an event marked by penetration of the ovum (female egg cell) by a spermatozoon (male germ cell). Conception results in a fertilized ovum. Only a fertilized ovum develops into a human being.

Answer	Frame
fertilization or conception	45. Penetration of the female egg cell by the male germ cell is known as ______________________.
ovum	46. Another term for female egg cell is ______________.
spermatozoon (sper′ ma tō zō′ on)	A term meaning male germ cell is ______________.
conception	47. Union of an ovum and a spermatozoon is called ______________.
fertilized	A child will develop from an ovum only if the ovum is ______________.
	Gestation is the period from conception to childbirth during which an ovum passes through several stages of development on the way to becoming a newborn infant. Gestation lasts 280 days from the last menstrual period.
pregnancy	48. Gestation is another word for the condition known as ______________.
gestation jes tā′ shun	Pregnancy is the condition of a female after conception until the birth of the baby. Pregnancy is another word for the period of time called ______________.
280	49. Gestation is the process of developing an ovum into a child. It takes ______________ days.
gestation pregnancy	50. An ovum develops into a child during a period from conception to birth. This process is called ______________ and the condition is called ______________.
gestation	51. During pregnancy an ovum passes through many developmental stages or phases. Taken together, these phases make up the nine-month period called ______________.
	The earliest gestational phase begins with a fertilized female egg cell. In just two weeks, the ovum divides into two cells, and each cell continues halving until it has become a complex mass of cells.

This mass of cells is now called an *embryo*. It's a living organism ready to continue its development into the next phase.

52.
The indispensable event that initiates a pregnancy is ________________.

conception

53.
After conception, the earliest phase of development begins with a fertilized ____________ and lasts ____________ weeks.

ovum
ō′ vum
two

54.
The first two weeks of gestation produce a complex living organism called a/an ____________.

embryo
em′ brē ō

The *embryo* begins a second stage of gestation in the third week, which lasts six weeks. In the third week, the embryo begins to acquire structure (head, arms, legs, and a tail), and over the next few weeks it begins forming principal internal organs and body systems. By the end of the eighth week of gestation the embryo looks somewhat like a human and is called a *fetus*.

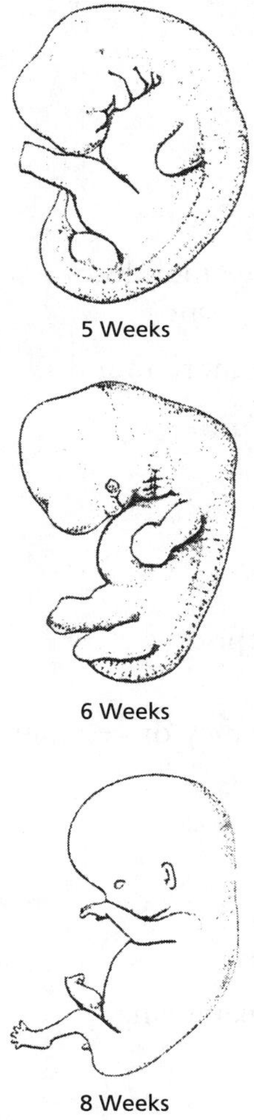

5 Weeks

6 Weeks

8 Weeks

Figure 9.3 Embryos at 5, 6, and 8 Weeks

55.
The second stage of gestation begins with a two-week-old ovum, which is now called an ____________.

embryo

56.
The embryo begins its second stage of development in the __________ week of gestation and continues through the ______________ week of a new pregnancy. At the beginning of the ninth week, it is called a ____________.

third
eighth
fetus

57.

During this second gestational phase the embryo begins forming arms and legs and principal internal ______________.

organs

58.

By the beginning of the ninth week, the embryo begins to resemble a ______________ and is called a ______________.

human being
fetus
fē′ tus

59.

A *fetus* begins the last phase of gestation. A fetus is a live offspring while it is in the mother (in utero). It continues developing during the remainder of the gestational period. The fetal stage lasts from the beginning of the third month of gestation to childbirth. A fetus sufficiently developed to sustain life outside the uterus is called a *viable* fetus.

In the last gestational phase, the fetus in utero develops into a ______________.

viable fetus

When does this phase begin? ______________

at three months of pregnancy

How long does it last? ______________

seven more months

What is the terminating event? ______________

childbirth

60.

Here's a quick review.

- Penetration of an ovum by a spermatozoon is called ______________.

conception

- A nine-month period during which a fertilized ovum becomes a child is called ______________.

pregnancy or gestation

- In the first two weeks of pregnancy an ovum becomes a complex organism called an ______________.

embryo

- From the third week to the beginning of the ninth week of pregnancy an embryo develops rudimentary appendages and internal ______________.

organs

- After only two months' gestation, the embryo begins to resemble ______________ and is called a ______________.

a human being
fetus

- A fetus developing in utero for the next seven months becomes a ______________.

human being or child

- Gestation ends with ______________.

childbirth

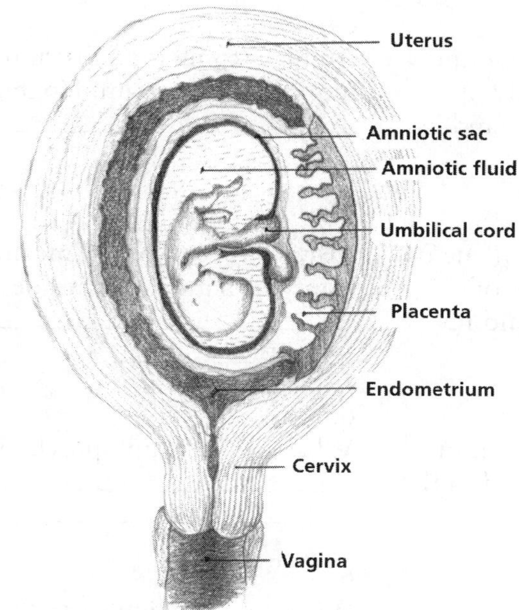

Figure 9.4. Fetus in Utero, Beginning 9th Week

uterus (hyster/o, metr/o)
amniotic sac (amni/o, amniot/o)
amniotic fluid (liquor amnii)

61.
Here are a few medical terms referring to some structures and conditions relating to pregnancy. *Amnion, amni/o, amniot/o* refer to a thin transparent sac containing the fetus and the fluid surrounding the fetus. This sac grows rapidly as the fetus inside develops. The amniotic fluid protects the fetus from injury and helps maintain an even temperature.

amniotic fluid
am nē ot′ ik flū′ id

Within the amniotic sac the fetus is protected from injury and changes in temperature by the *liquor amnii,* or in other words, ________________.

62.

amniotic

Amniot/itis means inflammation of the amnion. Build a word that means pertaining to the sac that envelops the fetus: ____________.

am′ nē ō sen tē′ sis
puncturing the amniotic sac and withdrawing some fluid

63.
The suffix *-centesis* means to puncture a cavity and remove fluid. Explain the meaning of amni/o/centesis: ______________________
____.

am′ nē ō tōm
usually an ultrasound graphic study of the amnion (and its contents)

64.
Amni/o/tome is an instrument for cutting (puncturing) the amnion. What does amni/ography mean? ______________________________

65.
ol′ i gō hī dram′ nē os
scanty amount of amniotic fluid in the sac

Olig-, oligo- is a prefix meaning little, small, scanty. Olig/uria means scanty urination. What does oligo/hydr/amnios mean? ______________________________

66.
excessive amount of amniotic fluid in the sac

What do you think polyhydramnios means? ______________________________

67.
amniotic sac or amnion

What structure envelops the fetus and contains the fluid protecting the fetus? ______________________________

68.
The *placenta* is a structure made up of a network of blood vessels (arteries and veins). The placenta makes an intimate bond with the inside lining of the uterus (endometrium), and attaches to the fetus by the umbilical cord. The fetus absorbs oxygen and nutrients from its mother through the placenta. The placenta and the uterus do not exchange blood, but transport oxygen and nutrients across a thin membrane. The fetus excretes carbon dioxide and other wastes through this same vascular structure. The placenta begins to form about the eighth day of gestation, and by the end of the pregnancy weighs about one-sixth the weight of the infant. After the birth of the child, the uterus expels the placenta and is sometimes called the *afterbirth*.

placenta

The fetus in utero absorbs oxygen and nutrients and excretes carbon dioxide and wastes through a vascular structure called the ____________________.

69.
1 pound
1 ounce

The placenta weighs one-sixth of the weight of the infant. If the baby's birth weight is 6 pounds, 6 ounces, what would you expect the placenta to weigh at the end of pregnancy? __________ pound __________ ounce.

en dō mē′ trē um the inside lining of the uterus	70. The placenta forms and grows on the endometrium and makes an intimate bond with it. What is the endometrium? ______________ ______________
placenta umbilical cord	71. While in utero the fetus grows by getting its nourishment through the ______________. The fetus is attached to the placenta by the ______________.
afterbirth	72. The placenta is expelled after the baby is born. The placenta is also called ______________.
pregnant (a current condition)	73. *Gravida, gravid* refers to a pregnant woman; being heavy with child. Gravidism is the condition of being ______________.
prī′ ma grav′ i da a woman who *is* pregnant with her first child	74. *Primi-* means first; *secundi-* means second. Primigravida refers to ______________ ______________.
a woman in her second pregnancy	What do you think gravida II means? ______________ ______________
secundigravida sē kun′ da grav′ i da	Build a compound medical term meaning a woman in her second pregnancy: ______________.
	75. Here's a quick review. From the suggested answers, select a term to go with each definition. Write your selection in the space provided.

SUGGESTED ANSWERS:

oligohydramnios	primigravida
amniocentesis	secundigravida
amniotic fluid	placenta

secundigravida	a woman in her second pregnancy ______________
primigravida	a pregnant woman, first time ______________
oligohydramnios	scanty fluid in the amnion ______________

	fetus in utero absorbs nutrients and excretes waste through it
placenta	________________
amniotic fluid	*liquor amnii* ________________
amniocentesis	puncture of the amnion and removal of fluid ________________

Labor and Delivery

Parturition is more commonly known as *labor.* Parturition is the process by which a baby is born and the placenta expelled from the uterus. This labor, or parturition, has three stages. The first stage is the stage of *dilation.* It is characterized by contractions of the uterine muscle and dilation of the birth canal and cervix—to let the baby out. The second stage is *expulsion.* The baby is born! In the third stage the placenta is expelled. This is the *placental* stage. The average duration of labor is about 13 hours in primagravida women (12 hours in dilation stage, 1 hour in expulsion stage, and a few minutes for the afterbirth). Labor is about 8 hours long in subsequent pregnancies.

76.
At term, when gestation is completed, a spontaneous physiological process begins. It has three stages: dilation, expulsion, and placental. This process is called ________________ or ________________.

Answer: parturition, labor

77.
In the first stage of labor, the uterus contracts rhythmically for 8 to 12 hours. The cervix thins and opens until it is fully dilated so the baby may pass through the birth canal. This first stage is called the ________________ stage.

Answer: dilation (dī lā′ shun)

78.
The second stage of labor involves expulsion. The infant passes through the birth canal and is ________________.

Answer: expelled, born

79.
Expulsion of the placenta follows the birth of the child. This stage of labor is known as the ________________ stage.

Answer: placental

80.
What happens during the expulsion stage, or the second stage of labor? ________________

Answer: a child is born (expelled)

81.
How long is the third stage of labor? ________

a few minutes

What happens in the placental stage of labor? ________

the placenta is expelled

82.
After 8 to 12 hours of uterine contractions during the first stage of labor, what has happened? ________

the cervix (neck of the uterus) completely dilates (opens)

83.
Parturition is another word for childbirth. What other term you just learned also means the process of being born? ________

par tyer ish′ un
labor

84.
Antepartum refers to the entire gestational period before labor begins.

What does postpartum mean? ________

after labor is completed

85.
Neo means new or recent. *Natus* is a Latin term for birth. What does neonatal mean? ________

the recent period around childbirth

86.
What do you think prenatal care means? ________

medical care and supervision of a pregnant woman before childbirth

87.
Review the terms you just learned before moving on. Select the term that best fits each brief definition. Use the suggestions if you need help.

labor	parturition
prenatal care	afterbirth
dilation	expulsion

medical supervision of a pregnant woman ________

prenatal care
prē nā′ tal kair

the process of giving birth ________

labor or parturition

parturition or labor	the act of childbirth ________
dilation	first stage of labor ________
expulsion	second stage of labor ________
placental	third stage of labor ________

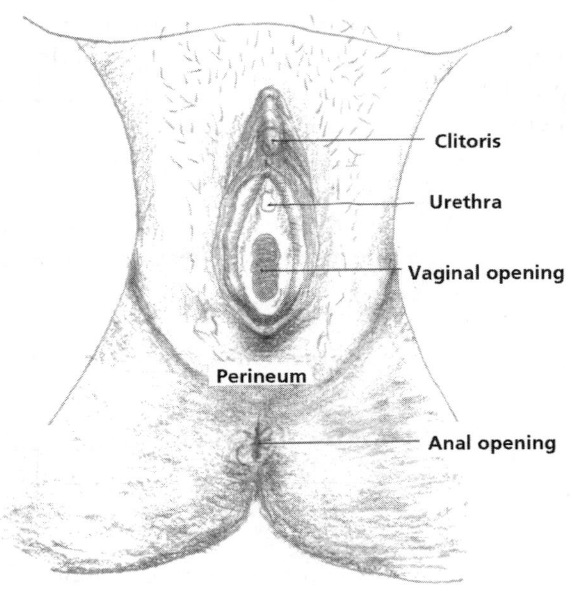

Figure 9.5. Female Pudenda

urethra (urethr/o) perineum
vagina (vagin/o) anus (an/o)

88.

Pudendum, pudenda (plural) means the external genitals (sex organs) of a female. These parts are easily observed without manual examination.

Take a look at Figure 9.5 above.

pudendal
pyo͞o den′ dl

Build a term meaning pertaining to the female's external genitals: ________________.

89.

Perineum refers to the structures that make up the pelvic outlet and comprise the pelvic floor. It is the region between the lip at the vaginal opening and anus in a female or between the scrotum and ______________ in a male.

anus
ā′ nus

90.
A baby coming through the birth canal during parturition can overstretch the vagina and the pelvic outlet. A tear (laceration) may occur in the tissues around the pelvic outlet. This pelvic floor structure is called the ____________________.

perineum
per i nē′ um

91.
Episiotomy is an incision of the perineum. During the second stage of labor, just before the baby is born, the obstetrician may incise the perineum to avoid fetal distress and subsequent hypoxia.

Episiotomy allows faster delivery of a distressed fetus and is an incision into the ____________________.

perineum

92.
What does episiorrhaphy mean? ____________________

suturing repair, reconstruction of the tissues after an episiotomy

93.
Here's a term often confused with perineum. *Peritoneum* is a tough membrane covering the viscera (organs in the belly) and lining the abdominal cavity. It clings to the viscera as plastic wrap clings to whatever it covers.

The membrane that coats the viscera and lines the abdominal cavity is the ____________________.
perineum/peritoneum

peritoneum
per i tō nē′ um

What is peritonitis? ____________________

per i tō nī′ tis
inflammation of the peritoneum

94.
Select the term that best fits the brief definition. Write it in the space provided.

peritoneum episiotomy
pudenda perineum

external female genitals ____________________

pudenda

the region of the external female genitals between the vaginal lip and anus ____________________

perineum

a membrane coating the viscera and lining the abdominal cavity ____________________

peritoneum

incision of the perineum to more quickly deliver a baby in distress

episiotomy ____________________

95.
Involution is a *process* the body goes through that reduces the uterus to its normal nonpregnant size and condition following childbirth.

The process that returns an enlarged uterus to its normal size after the baby is born is called ____________________.

involution

96.
Puerperium is a *period of time* following the third stage of labor when involution takes place. Involution lasts approximately six weeks.

pōō er pēr′ ē um

Puerperium begins after the fetus and the placenta have been ____________________.

expelled

97.
Puerperium lasts until the uterus returns to its size and condition before pregnancy began. This period of time is approximately ____________ weeks.

six

98.
After fulfilling its function, the uterus goes through a process of returning to its earlier nonpregnant condition. This process is called ____________________.

involution

99.
Involution takes place during a six-week period after childbirth. This time period is called the ____________________.

puerperium
pōō er pēr′ ē um

100.
Explain the meaning of the term puerperal. ____________________
____
____

of or pertaining to the period after childbirth when involution takes place

101.
Sepsis means the presence of pathogenic organisms or bacteria that have entered the bloodstream and cause serious infections. Years ago, prior to effective antibiotic therapy, the greatest single cause of death following childbirth was called *childbed fever.*

Another description of this condition is ____________________ sepsis.
(pertaining to the time when involution takes place)

puerperal (sepsis)

inflammation of the peritoneum during puerperium	102. What is puerperal peritonitis? ______________________________
the process by which the uterus returns to its earlier nonpregnant state after childbirth	103. Involution takes place during puerperium. What does involution mean? ______________________________
nulli/para nullipara nu lip′ ə ra	104. *Nulli-* is a prefix meaning none. *Para* means to bear a child. Build a term that refers to a woman who has never borne a child: ______________ / ____________.
prīm ip′ ə ra a woman who has given birth to one viable child (an event in the past)	105. A woman who has delivered more than one living child is described as *multipara.* What does *primipara* mean? ______________________________
she has given birth to two viable children	106. What does an obstetrician mean when he writes in the patient's chart that she is para-2? ______________________________
	107. Using the word root *para* and *nulli-, multi-,* or *primi-,* build a word for each of the following abbreviations.
primipara nullipara multipara mul tip′ ə ra	para-1 ____________________ para-0 ____________________ para-4 ____________________
	108. It's a good time to review what you just covered. Select a term from the suggestions and complete each brief definition.
	nullipara parturition primigravida antepartum involution puerperium
involution	the process taking place after childbirth that reduces the uterus to normal size and condition ____________________

puerperium	the six-week period after childbirth when involution takes place ______________
antepartum	the period in a pregnancy occurring before labor ______________
nullipara	a woman who has never given birth to a viable child ______________
primigravida	a woman who is pregnant for the first time ever ______________
parturition	another term for labor ______________

109.
Here are some terms you may find very interesting. Look them up. You'll be surprised at how much you have learned.

acquired
anomaly
placenta abruptio
congenital
eclampsia
placenta previa

110.
Here are 50 new words you worked with in this unit. When you pronounce each term be sure to think about what it means. Then take the Chapter 9 Self-Test.

amenorrhea (ä men ō rē′ a)
amniocentesis (am′ nē ō sen tē′ sis)
amnion (am′ nē on)
amniotic fluid (am nē ôt ik flo͞o′ id)
climacteric (klī mak′ ter ik)
conception (kon sep′ shun)
dysmenorrhea (dis men ōr ē′ ə)
embryo
endometrium (en′ dō mē′ trē um)
episiotomy (e pēz ē ot′ ō mē)
fetus
gestation (jes tā′ shun)
gynecomastia (gī′ ne kō mas′ tē ə)
gynoplasty (jin′ ō plas tē)
hysterocele (his′ ter ō sēl)
hysteromyoma (his′ ter ō mī ō′ mä)
hysterorrhexis (his′ ter ō rek′ sis)
involution (in vō lo͞o′ shun)
labor
mammalgia (ma mal′ jē ə)
mammary (mam′ ə rē)
mammopexy (mam′ ō pek sē)
mastodynia (mas tō din′ ē ə)
mastoncus (mas tong′ kus)
mastopathy (mas top′ ə thē)
mastoptosis (mas top tō′ sis)
menometrorrhagia (men′ ō mētrō rā′ jē ə)
menopause (men′ ō pawz)
menorrhalgia (men ō ral′ jē ə)
menses (men′ sēz)
menstruation (men strū ā′ shun)

metratrophy (mē tra′ trō fē)
metrorrhagia (mē trō ra′ jē ə)
multipara (mul tip′ ə ra)
myometritis (mī′ ō mē trī′ tis)
neonatal (nē ō nā′ tal)
nullipara (nu lip′ ə ra)
oligohydramnios
(ol′ ē gō hī dram′ nē ōs)
ovum (ō′ vum)
parturition (pär tyo͞or ish′ un)
perineum (per i nē′ um)
peritoneum (per i tō nē′ um)
placenta
polyhydramnios
(pä lē hī dram′ nē ōs)
postpartum
primigravida
(prī′ ma grav′ i da)
pudenda (pyo͞o den′ də)
puerperal sepsis
(po͞o er′ per al sep sis)
puerperium
(po͞o er pēr′ ē um)
spermatozoon
(sper′ ma tō zō′ on)

Chapter 9 Self-Test

Part 1

From the right, select the correct meaning for each of the following medical terms.

______ 1. Primigravida
______ 2. Pudenda
______ 3. Hysteropathy
______ 4. Mammary
______ 5. Mastrodynia
______ 6. Amniotic
______ 7. Episiotomy
______ 8. Endometritis
______ 9. Involution
______ 10. Metratrophy
______ 11. Perineum
______ 12. Amenorrhea
______ 13. Puerperium
______ 14. Hysterorrhexis
______ 15. Mammography

a. X ray study of the breast
b. Temporary lack of menstruation
c. Pelvic floor, region from vaginal lip to anus
d. Process of returning uterus to nonpregnant state
e. Incision of vagina and pelvic outlet
f. Female external genitals
g. Pregnant woman, first time
h. Period after childbirth, when involution takes place
i. Pertaining to sac holding the fetus and fluid
j. Rupture of uterus (during labor)
k. Pertaining to the breast
l. Uterine atrophy (wasting)
m. Inflammation of uterine inside lining
n. Painful breasts
o. Uterine disease

Part 2

Write the medical term for each of the following brief definitions.

1. Surgical fixation of pendulous breasts ______
2. Membrane covering abdominal viscera (organs) ______
3. Painful breasts ______
4. Change-of-life period Female ______
5. Organism in utero resembling a human ______
6. Organ that nourishes fetus in utero ______
7. Surgical removal of the breast ______
8. Another term for pregnancy ______
9. Pertaining to a recently born child ______
10. Woman pregnant with her first child ______
11. Pendulous breast ______
12. Fertilization of an ovum ______
13. Labor and delivery of term pregnancy ______
14. Pertaining to before the onset of labor ______
15. After childbirth when involution takes place P ______

ANSWERS

Part 1	*Part 2*
1. g	1. Mammopexy
2. f	2. Peritoneum
3. o	3. Mastodynia, mammalgia
4. k	4. Female climacteric
5. n	5. Fetus
6. i	6. Placenta
7. e	7. Mastectomy
8. m	8. Gestation
9. d	9. Neonatal

10. l	10. Primipara
11. c	11. Mastoptosis
12. b	12. Conception
13. h	13. Parturition
14. j	14. Antepartum
15. a	15. Puerperium

10 The Eye

In this chapter you'll work with new terms relating to the eye along with other areas in close proximity, including the nose and throat. You will use some new word roots and combining forms and put them together with many suffixes you are already familiar with.

This section of the head to toe assessment is known as HEENT, which stands for head, eyes, ears, nose, and throat. As you learn new medical terms, note the words that might fall into HEENT and remember back to Chapters 2 and 3 when you learned the basic medical terms including many involving this section of the assessment. These data will provide information on the patient's neurological status (how well the nerves are working), sensory status (whether those nerves are transmitting good signals to the brain about touch and temperature), and any malformations or indications of congenital anomalies (conditions a person is born with). Remember also that the sensory assessment includes a visual exam (to determine how well the eyes see, move, and respond to certain stimuli), a hearing test (to determine how well the ear transmits sounds), a smell assessment (to determine how well the nose transmits smells), and a taste evaluation (to determine how well the tongue transmits taste). The last part of this section is for assessing the throat, including all the lymph nodes, the parts of the respiratory tract contained in the throat, the blood vessels inside the throat, and the thyroid. To get started, review the mini-glossary below.

Mini-Glossary

Root Words

blephar/o (*eyelid*)
core, core/o (*pupil*)
corne/o, kerat/o (*cornea*)
cycl/o (*ciliary body*)
dipl/o (*paired, double*)
ir, irid/o (*iris*)
lacrim/o (*tear*)
ophthalm/o (*eye*)
retin/o (*retina*)
scler/o (*sclera*)

Don't forget to complete the Review Sheet for Chapter 9 before beginning Chapter 10. Keep up the good work!

1.

Let's refresh your memory. You'll find it helpful to review suffixes you already studied and will use again in the first section. Write the meaning of each of the following. Do your best without looking at the answers.

Answer	Suffix
twitching	-spasm ________
suturing, repair	-orrhaphy ________
inflammation of	-itis ________
a diseased condition	-pathy ________
instrument that cuts	-tome ________
dilation, stretching	-ectasia ________
resembling, like	-oid ________
to fix, fixation (into normal place)	-pexy ________
pertaining to out of normal place	-ectopic ________
hernia, herniation	-cele ________
drooping, prolapse	-ptosis ________
measuring, measuring instrument	metr-, -meter ________
instrument for examining, looking inside of	-scope, -scopy ________
treatment, treating a condition	-therapy ________
surgery to restore or make new	-plasty ________

2.
Now, let's try it the other way. Write the suffix that satisfies the definition given in the table below. Then check your answers. You may want to use this table to help you complete the next few frames.

Answer	Definition	Suffix
-metr, -meter	to measure, instrument for measuring	______
-therapy	treatment for a condition	______
-itis	inflammation of	______
-ectasia	dilation, stretch	______
-ptosis	drooping, prolapse	______
-scope, -scopy	examine, instrument to look inside	______
-plasty	surgery to restore, make new	______
-oid	resembling, like	______
-spasm	twitching	______
-pathy	a diseased condition	______
-pexy	surgically fix into normal place	______
-orrhaphy	suture, repair after trauma	______
-tome	instrument for cutting	______
-ectopic	pertaining to out of normal place	______
-cele	hernia, rupture	______

The Eye

of, pertaining to, or relating to the eye

opthalm-

ophthalm/o

3.
Here are some new terms. Ophthalmology is the medical specialty concerned with the eye and its diseases. Ophthalm/o/malacia means an abnormal softening of the eyeball.
What is the word root? ______________
Write the combining form: ______________.

of

of thal′ mō

4.
Ophthalm, ophthalm/o are the word root and combining form for terms difficult to spell and pronounce. But if you pronounce the words correctly, the spelling will be easier. For example, oph/thal/mo is pronounced of thal′ mō. The oph is pronounced as ________.
In the word root ophthalm-, ph comes before th, as in the alphabet (p before t). Oph thal mō is pronounced ______________.
Pronounce it.

5.
Here's a chance to practice your spelling and pronunciation. Use the combining form ophthalm/o and add each of these suffixes to build new words.

-cele	hernia, herniation
-meter	instrument for measuring
-plegia	paralysis

Build a term and then pronounce it carefully:

ophthalmocele
of thal′ mō sēl

herniation of the eye (abnormal protrusion) ____________________

ophthalmometer
of′ thal mom′ e ter

instrument for measuring the eye ____________________

ophthalmoplegia
of thal′ mo plē′ gē a

paralysis of the eye (eye muscle) ____________________

ophthalmologist
of thal mol′ ō jist

6.
The physician who practices the medical specialty concerned with diseases of the eye is an ____________________.

ophthalmoscope
of thal′ mō skōp

7.
The instrument used for examining the interior of the eyeball through the pupil is an ____________________.

double vision

8.
Dipl/o means double or paired. -*Opia* is a suffix meaning vision. What does dipl/opia mean? ____________________

diplopia
di plō′ pē a

9.
Whenever a pair of eyes fail to record a singular image in the brain, a double image occurs. The medical term for double vision is ____________________.

10.
Write a brief meaning for each of the following.

double (or paired) bacteria

dipl/o/bacteria ____

bluish vision

cyan/opia ____________________

11.

blef a rop′ tō sis
blephar-
blephar/o

Blephar/optosis means prolapse (drooping) of an eyelid. The word root for eyelid is ________________. The combining form is ________________.

12.

blef ar e dē′ ma
blephar<u>edema</u>

Blephar/edema means excess fluid in the tissues of the eyelid. Underline the part of the term meaning swelling due to fluid in the tissues: blepharedema.

13.

blepharedema

The condition of swollen eyelids due to excess fluid in the eyelids is ________________.

14.

Define each of the following terms:

blef′ ar ō spazm
twitching of the eyelid

Blepharospasm means ________________________________ ________________.

blef ar ōr′ a fē
suturing of the eyelid

Blepharorrhaphy means ________________________________ ________________.

15.

blef ar ī′ tis
blepharitis

Build a word that means inflammation of the eyelid: ________________.

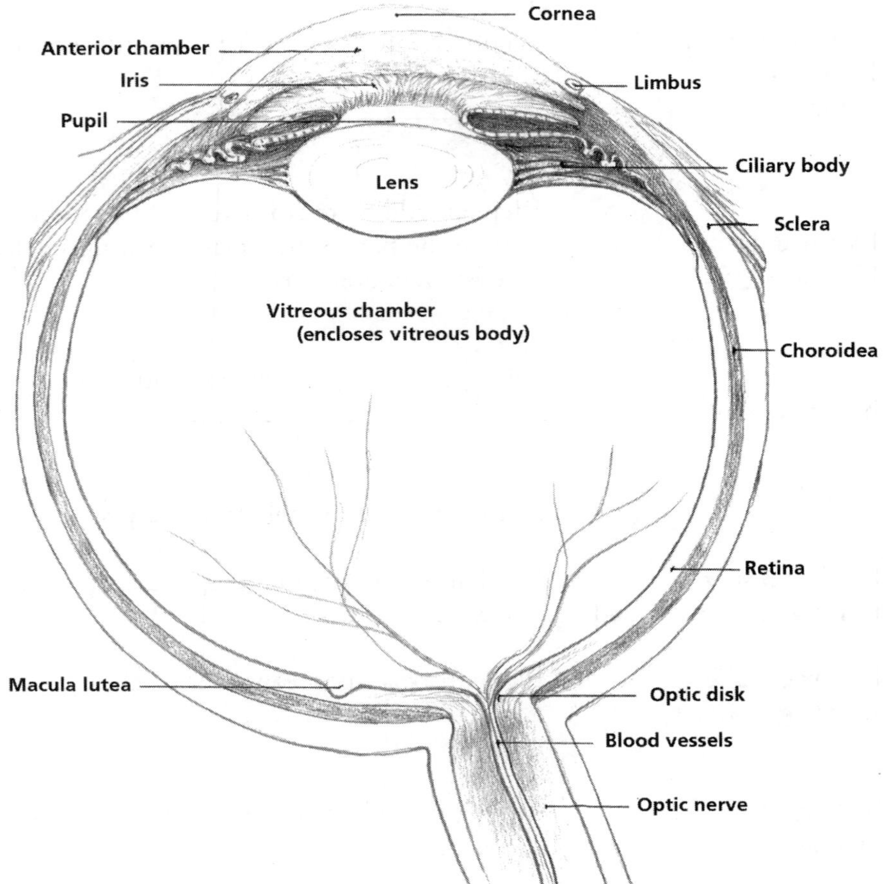

Figure 10.1 The Eye

Sight is the most dominant of the human senses. Over 70% of the body's receptors are the specialized photosensitive cells of the eyes. It has been estimated that a third of all the fibers bringing impulses to the central nervous system come from the eye. The eye is also a window into brain function and can be an important indicator of disturbances in the brain.

The human eye is somewhat like a camera that captures light and focuses it on a light-sensitive area. The wall of the eyeball consists of three coats or layers of tissue. The first layer is the fibrous, rubberlike protective coat called the *sclera,* known as the white of the eye. The sclera gives the eyeball its shape, and can be seen around most of the eyeball's surface. A continuation of the sclera and the most anterior segment of this fibrous coat is the cornea. The *cornea* is a transparent structure that bulges and has no blood vessels. It plays a big role in focusing light rays on the retina of the eye. The area called the *limbus* is where the cornea meets the sclera.

The middle layer of the eyeball is the vascular layer called the *choroidea.* It lies between the retinal and the scleral layers. The choroidea contains many blood vessels and includes the iris and the ciliary body. The iris, or the colored part of the eye seen through the cornea, is a fibromuscular body that circumscribes the hole (pupil) in front of the lens. Action of the iris increases and decreases the size of the pupil. Another portion of the choroidea is the ciliary body. This structure is continuous with the iris and contains the ciliary muscle, which controls eye movement. The lens is a tightly packed and encapsulated bunch of special fibers. Along with the cornea, it shares responsibility for bringing images into focus on the retina.

The fluid-filled space between the iris and the cornea is the *anterior chamber.* It contains a fluid material called aqueous humor that services the cells within its environment. A large cavity posterior to the lens is known as the *vitreous chamber.* This cavity contains a clear, gelatinous mass known as the vitreous body. The vitreous body maintains the shape of the eye and gives support to the retina.

The *retina* is the innermost coat of the eye, the neural layer. It lines a bit more than the posterior half of the globe. The retina is a complexly composed network of interlacing layers of blood vessels and photoreceptor cells that come together at the *optic disk.* This is actually a blind spot since there are no photoreceptors here. The optic disk penetrates the wall of the eye and forms the optic nerve, which carries impulses to the brain.

When light enters the eye, it passes through the cornea, pupil, and lens, and focuses an image on the retina. At about the center of the retina there is a clearly depressed region with a dense accumulation of photoreceptor cells. This area of the retina providing the sharpest vision is called the *macula lutea.* At the center of macula is the *fovea centralis.* This site represents the center of the greatest visual acuity (clarity of form and color) under lighted conditions.

I hope you enjoyed your tour of the anatomy of the eye.

cornea (kerat/o)	sclera (skler/o)
iris (ir, irid, irid/o)	pupil (cor, core/o)
retina (retin/o)	ciliary body (cycl/o)

16.

Use Figure 10.1, The Eye, and the accompanying description. The cornea is the transparent tissue covering the anterior sixth of the eye. *Kerat, kerat/o* form words referring to the cornea. Write the meaning of each of the following:

kor nē a
the transparent tissue covering the anterior sixth of the eye

cornea ______________________________

ker a top′ a thē
disease of the cornea

kerat/o/pathy ______________________________

17.

keratoplasty
ker′ a tō plas tē

Using the combining form kerat/o, build a term meaning plastic repair of the cornea: ____________.

18.

kerat, kerat/o

The cornea is one-sixth of the outer coat of the eyeball. It is the transparent tissue covering the front of the eyeball. The word root and combining form meaning cornea are ____________.

19.

cornea

Scler/o refers to the white of the eye. The sclera is the hard fibrous coat forming the outer envelope of the eye. It covers five-sixths of the eyeball. The other anterior sixth is occupied by the ____________.

20.

Corneoscleral means pertaining to an area where the cornea meets the sclera. Write the meaning for each of the following:

skler′ al
pertaining to the sclera

scleral ______________________________
____

skler′ ō tōm
instrument for cutting the sclera

sclerotome ______________________________
____

21.

sclerectomy
skle rek′ tō mē

Sclerectasia means bulging (stretching) of the white of the eye. Build a term meaning excision of a portion of the sclera:
____________.

ī′ ris
ir′ i dō kor′ nē al
pertaining to the area where the iris and cornea meet

22.
Iris means rainbow. The iris is a diaphragm perforated in the center (the pupil). The word roots referring to the donut-shaped color in the eye are *ir, irid,* and *irid/o*. What do you think iridocorneal mea ns? ____

ir′ id ō sēl
hernia of the iris

Iridocele means ____.

ir/itus
iritis
ī rī′ tis

23.
One of the word roots for the iris is ir. It has very limited use, but it's always used to express inflammation.

Using the word root ir build a word meaning inflammation of the iris: ________ / ______________.

i ri dal′ jē ə
pain in the iris

24.
Irid/o is the combining form used to refer to the iris in almost all other words. Iridalgia means ______________________________.

iridectomy
i ri dek′ tō mē

25.
Build a term meaning excision of part of the iris: ____________________.

cornea
vision, sight
iris
sclera
eye
eyelid
iris

26.
Write what each of the following word roots or combining forms means.

kerat/o ____________________
opia ____________________
irid/o ____________________
scler/o ____________________
ophthalm/o ____________________
blephar/o ____________________
ir ____________________

retinal
ret′ i n'l
retinitis
ret i nī′ tis
retinoid
ret′ i noyd

27.
Retin/o refers to the complex membrane lining the inside back surface of the eye. It receives the visual light rays, which the brain interprets and gives meaning. Build a word meaning

pertaining to the retina ____________________

inflammation of the retina ____________________

resembling the retina ____________________

28.
Retinopexy means affixing (or adhering) the retina to the wall of the eyeball for correcting retinal detachment. What would you call an instrument for examining the retina to look for retinopathy?
____

retinoscope or ophthalmoscope
ret′ i nō skōp

29.
What does retinopathy mean? ________________

ret i nop′ a thē
disease of the retina

30.
The pupil is the circular opening in the center of the iris through which the light rays enter the eye. It is the core or center of the eye. *Cor, core/o* refer to the pupil in the center of the ________.

(eye), iris

31.
An ophthalmologist may use drops in the eye to dilate the pupil before an examination.

Analyze the term cor/ectasia.

Cor- is the root meaning ________;

ectasia means ________.

What does cor/ectopia mean? ________________

pupil
dilation
kōr ek tō′ pē a
a misplaced pupil

32.
Coreoplasty is a surgical procedure for correcting a deformed pupil.

Write a term meaning to measure the size of a pupil. ________________

kōr ē om′ e trē
coreometry

33.
Take another look at Figure 10.1, The Eye. The ciliary body controls movement of the eye. The word root for ciliary body is *cycl/o*. It means circle or surrounding.

What does cyclo/paralysis mean? ________________

sī klō pa ral′ i sis
paralysis of the ciliary body

34.
Cyclocryotherapy means freezing of the ciliary body in the treatment of glaucoma. Underline the part of the term referring to freezing: cyclocryotherapy.

sī klō krī′ ō ther′ a pē
cyclo<u>cryo</u>therapy

sī klō ker a tī′ tis
inflammation of the cornea and the ciliary body

35.
Use Figure 10.1 for help. Cyclitis means inflammation of the ciliary body. What is the meaning of cyclokeratitis? ______________________
____
____

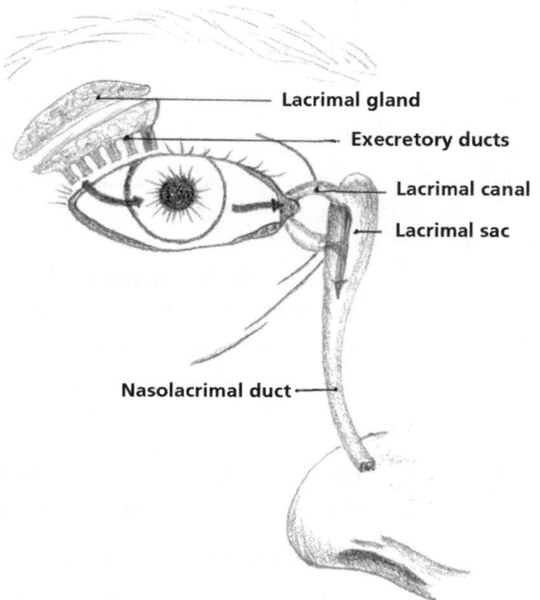

Figure 10.2 The Lacrimal Apparatus

The human lacrimal apparatus is responsible for producing tears and delivering them to the eye. When an excess is produced, the tears flow into the nasal cavities.

The lacrimal apparatus begins with the *lacrimal gland* seen under the upper lateral eyebrow and extending inward toward the mid-line. Blinking stimulates the lacrimal gland to secrete lacrimal fluid (tears), which wash the eye. It also contains substances that destroy the cell walls of bacteria, and it moistens the surface of the eye. The fluid passes through a series of excretory ducts and enters a fold of tissue under the upper eyelid. The eyelid then distributes the tears across the eyeball. Excess fluid flows to the medial corner of the eye passing through a tiny opening and entering the *lacrimal canal.* The upper and lower lacrimal canals drain into the *lacrimal sac.* Excess tears move from the lacrimal sac into the *nasolacrimal duct* and pass through an opening into the nose. This is the reason one sniffles when crying.

36.
Look again at Figure 10.2. The lacrimal apparatus consists of the gland, the sac, and the duct. The purpose of the lacrimal apparatus is to keep the surface of the eye moist and protected. What do you think lacrimal means? ________________

lak′ ri mal
relating to tears

37.
The gland that secretes tears is the ________________ gland.

lacrimal

The sac that collects the tears is the ________________ sac.

lacrimal

What is the structure that empties the tears into the nasal cavity?
________________ ________

nasolacrimal duct

38.
Tears keep the surface of the eye moistened. Tears are continually being formed and removed. When tears form more quickly than they can be removed by the lacrimal apparatus, we say the person is ________________.

crying

39.
How about a review? Complete each of the following brief definitions. Use the suggested answers to help you.

SUGGESTED ANSWERS:

iritis	cycloplegia
lacrimal	diplopia
cyclocryotherapy	sclerotome
retinoscopy	ophthalmic
coreometry	keratitis
iridocele	keratoplasty

measurement of pupil size ________________
herniation of the iris ________________
pertaining to the eye ________________
examination of the retina ________________
inflammation of the iris ________________
instrument for cutting the sclera ________________
relating to tears ________________
surgical reconstruction of the cornea ________________
paralytic ciliary body ________________
inflammation of the cornea ________________
double vision ________________
treatment (of glaucoma) freezing the ciliary body
____

coreometry
iridocele
ophthalmic
retinoscopy
iritis
sclerotome
lacrimal
keratoplasty
cycloplegia
keratitis
diplopia
cyclocryotherapy

40.
Try these now. Write the meaning of each of the following word roots:

Answer	Word root
retina	retin/o ______________
pupil	cor/o, core/o ______________
ciliary body	cycl/o ______________
eyelid	blephar/o ______________
cornea	kerat/o (corne/o) ______________
eye	ophthalm/o ______________
sight, vision	opia ______________
iris	irid/o ______________

41.
Here are 27 more medical terms you have worked with in Chapter 10. Don't forget to pronounce each one carefully before taking the final Chapter 10 Self-Test.

blepharedema (blef′ ar ə dē′ mä)
blepharorrhaphy (blef ar ōr′ ā fē)
blepharoptosis (blef ar op tō′ sis)
corectasia (kōr ek tā′ zē ə)
corectopia (kōr ek tō′ pē ə)
coreometer (kōr ē om′ e ter)
coreoplasty (kōr′ ē ō plas tē)
corneal (kor′ nē al)
cyclokeritits (sī′ klō ker i tī′ tis)
cycloplegia (sī klō plē′ jē ə)
diplopia (di plō′ pē ə)
iridectomy (ir i dek′ tō mē)
iridocele (ir id ō sēl)
iridoplegia (ir id ō plē′ jē ə)
iritis (ī rī′ tis)
keratome (ker′ ə tōm)
keratoplasty (ker′ ə tō plas tē)
keratoscleritis (ker′ ə tō skler ī′ tis)
keratotomy (ker a tōt′ ō mē)
nasolacrimal (nā zō lak′ ri məl)
ophthalmalgia (of′ thal mal′ jē a)
ophthalmoscope (of thal′ mō skōp)
retinitis (ret i nī′ tis)
retinopathy (ret i nop′ ə thē)
retinoscopy (ret i nos′ kō pē)
sclerectomy (skler ek′ tō mē)
sclerotome (skler′ ə tōm)

Chapter 10 Self-Test

Part 1

From the list on the right, select the correct meaning for each of the following often used medical terms.

______	1. Keratoscleritis	a. Stretching (dilation) of the pupil
______	2. Corectasia	b. Instrument to cut the cornea
______	3. Blepharedema	c. Paralysis of the iris
______	4. Ophthalmologist	d. Inflammation of cornea and sclera
______	5. Iridoplegia	e. Resembling the retina
______	6. Keratome	f. Swollen eyelids due to fluid in the tissues
______	7. Retinoid	g. Physician who specializes in the study of eye diseases

Part 2

Write the medical term for each of the following brief definitions.

1. Pertaining to nose and tears ______________________
2. Instrument to examine the eye ______________________
3. Plastic surgery of the cornea ______________________
4. Double vision ______________________
5. Drooping eyelid ______________________
6. Inflammation of the iris ______________________
7. Pertaining to the cornea ______________________

ANSWERS

Part 1	***Part 2***
1. d	1. Nasolacrimal
2. a	2. Ophthalmoscope
3. f	3. Keratoplasty
4. g	4. Diplopia
5. c	5. Blepharoptosis
6. b	6. Iritis
7. e	7. Corneal

11 The Respiratory Tract

In Chapter 11 you'll work on new terms relating to the respiratory tract. Some words will be familiar; others are new. Practice your compound medical terms as you learn new root words throughout this chapter.

Chapter 11 rounds out our head-to-toe assessment with the respiratory system. Respiratory provides information about how a patient is breathing and about the effectiveness of oxygen exchange. Assessment includes sounds listened to with a stethoscope over the lungs, an inspection assessment to look for abnormalities, a percussion (tapping) assessment to listen for abnormalities, and a palpation (touching) assessment to feel for abnormalities. This combination of techniques can tell us if the lungs are working effectively, and it provides information for the head-to-toe assessment. Review the mini-glossary below to get started on Chapter 11.

Mini-Glossary

Root Words

bronch/i (*bronch/o, bronchus*)
laryng/o (*voice box*)
ment/o (*chin*)
nas/o (*nose*)
pharyng/o (*throat*)
pleur/o (*covering of the lung*)
pne/o (*air, breathe*)
pneum/o (*air, breathe*)
pneumon/o (*lung*)
thorac/o (*thorax*)
trache/o (*windpipe*)

Don't forget to complete the Review Sheet for Chapter 10 before beginning Chapter 11. Keep up the good work!

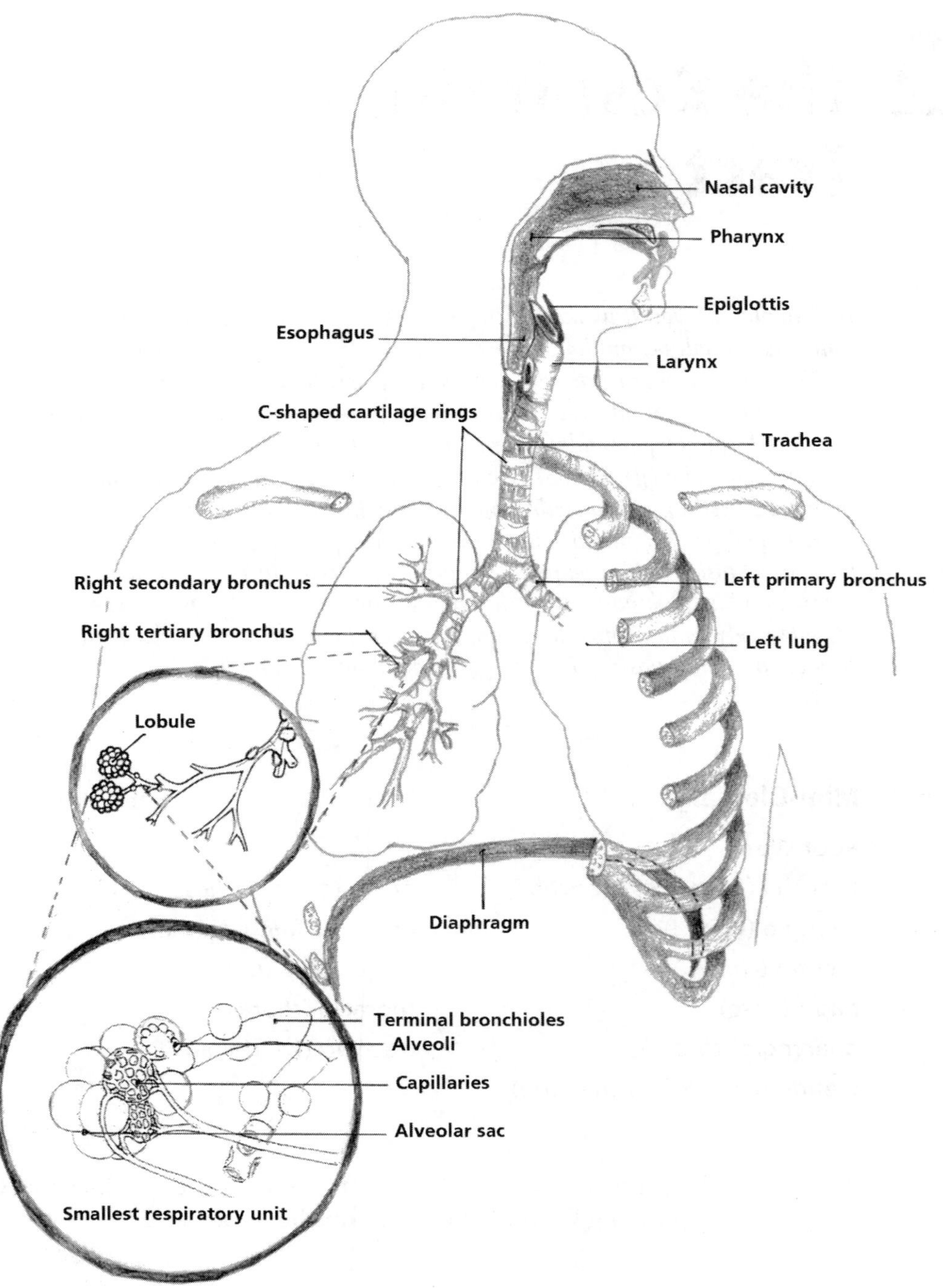

Figure 11.1 The Respiratory Tract (Cutaway Views)

The respiratory system consists of passageways that receive incoming air and carry it to the *lungs* for exchange of oxygen and carbon dioxide gases. The lungs are the main organs of gas exchange in the body. They are soft, spongy organs enveloped in a tough, wet and slippery transparent membrane called the *pleura.* The lungs are protected by the bony cage of the thorax. Most of the rest of the skeleton of the respiratory tract is cartilaginous, right down to the smallest air passageway. The dome-shaped muscular *diaphragm* provides most of the force necessary for inspiration and expiration of air. One quarter of the force is generated by the intercostal muscles moving the ribs. When the diaphragm contracts and flattens in its space, air enters the lungs. When it relaxes, air is expelled from the lungs. The diaphragm is the primary muscle in respiration.

Air enters the respiratory tract through the oral and nasal cavities. The *nasal cavity* houses the olfactory sense organ used in the sense of smell. The *pharynx* is an open area continuous with the nasal cavity, and its lower end opens to the *esophagus* and *larynx.* These upper passageways warm, moisten, and purify the air on its way to the lower respiratory tract.

The *larynx* is an enlarged section of the upper respiratory tract at the top of the trachea. The opening to the larynx is guarded by a leaf-like flap of cartilage called the *epiglottis.* This structure prevents food from entering the respiratory passageway and directs it to the esophagus. Beneath the epiglottis is the opening to the larynx called the *glottis.* The larynx houses the vocal cords, an important component of the larynx used in speaking. For this reason, the larynx is often called the voice box. The vocal cords are composed of elastic fibers that help produce sound when air is forced between them. These sound waves are formed into words by the changing shapes of the pharynx and oral cavity and by using the tongue and lips.

Inferior to the larynx is the *trachea,* the passageway of air to the lungs. The trachea is a flexible cylindrical tube about one inch in diameter and approximately four inches in length. It is composed of 16 to 20 incomplete c-shaped rings of cartilage connected to one another by very elastic ligaments. The cartilage rings provide a semi-rigid support to the wall of the trachea, preventing it from collapsing inward. The trachea extends downward in front of the esophagus and into the thoracic cavity.

The *bronchial tree* consists of the branched airways extending from the trachea to the smallest respiratory unit in the lung. It begins with the left and right *primary bronchi* (pl.). Each primary bronchus enters a lung and then subdivides, forming left and right *secondary bronchi.* We see three secondary bronchi in the anatomical right lung. The secondary bronchi branch again and the *tertiary bronchi* become *bronchioles,* less than 1 mm in diameter. These bronchioles give off smaller *terminal bronchioles* that represent the end of the air-conducting pathway.

Each *respiratory bronchiole* supplies air to lobules. A lobule is a basic gas exchange complex composed of air cells, called *alveoli,* which are arranged in *alveolar sacs.* The alveoli are arranged in grapelike clusters. The walls of the air cells are surrounded by capillaries. *Capillaries* are networks of pulmonary *arterioles* and pulmonary *venules.* The walls of the capillaries are fused to the structurally similar walls of the alveoli. Oxygen and carbon dioxide rapidly diffuse through the walls of these microscopic cells. The blood readily absorbs the oxygen and gives up the carbon dioxide, which is quickly exhausted to the external atmosphere. These basic units make up most of the lung's volume. The respiratory system is considered relatively sterile and therefore well protected. Nowhere in the body does the outside world, with all its creatures of microscopic dimension, have such an easy access to the protected interior cavities of the body as it does at the air/blood interfaces in the lungs.

lung (pneumon/o)
nasal cavity (nas/o)
esophagus (esophag/o)
breathe, breathing (pne/o)
trachea (trache/o)
bronchus, (bronch/o), whether primary, secondary, or tertiary parts of the bronchial tree
diaphragm
pharynx (pharyng/o)
larynx (laryng/o)
air, gases (pneum/o)
pleura (pleur/o)

1.
Pne/o comes from the Greek word *pneia* (breathe). Pne/o anyplace in a word means ________________.

breathe or breathing

2.
When pne/o begins a word, the "p" is silent. When pne/o occurs later in a word, the "p" is pronounced; for example, when you pronounce brady/pnea, you __________ (will/will not) pronounce the letter "p."
In the term pneumonia, the "p" is ______________ (pronounced/silent).

will
brad ip nē′ ə
silent

3.
Brady/pnea means ______________.

slow breathing

tachy/pnea
tachypnea
tak ip nē′ ə

A word for rapid breathing is ______________ / ________.

4.

tachypnea

The rate of respiration (breathing) is controlled by the amount of carbon dioxide in the blood. Increased carbon dioxide speeds up breathing and causes ____________________.

5.

tachypnea

Muscle exercise increases the amount of carbon dioxide in the blood. This speeds respiration and produces ____________________.

6.

without breathing

The prefix *a*- literally means without. Thus apnea means __________ ______________________________.

7.

apnea
ap′ nē ə

A/pnea really means temporary cessation of breathing. If the failure to breathe were not temporary, death would result. Temporary cessation of breathing is referred to as ___________.

8.

apnea
a-

If the level of carbon dioxide in the blood falls very low, temporary cessation of breathing results. This is called ________________. The prefix meaning without is _____.

9.

bradypnea

If breathing is merely very slow, it is called ____________________.

10.

tachypnea

When breathing is abnormally fast, it is called ____________________.

11.

See above to help you identify the word root for each anatomical part. Then write a meaning for each of the following terms.

la rin jī′ tis
inflammation of the voice box

laryng/itis ____ ______________________________.

plo͞or ī′ tis
inflammation of the pleura

pleuritis ____ ______________________________.

fair ing′ gō plas tē
plastic surgery of the throat

pharyng/o/plasty ____ ______________________________.

12.
Look again at Figure 11.1. Seeing the various parts will help you learn. What does laryng/o/cele mean? ____________________
____

la ring′ gō sēl
herniation of the voice box

13.
Build a term meaning surgical removal of the voice box:
__________________.

laryngectomy
la rin jek′ tō mē

14.
Write a meaning for each of the following:

laryngoscope ____
____

la ring′ gō skōp
instrument for examining the voice box

laryngospasm ____
____

la ring′ gō spazm
spasm of the voice box

15.
See Figure 11.1 again. *Trachea* means windpipe. Write a brief definition for each of the following new terms:

tracheorrhagia ____
____

trā kē ō rā′ jē ə
hemorrhage from the windpipe

trachealgia ____
____

trā kē al′ jē ə
pain in the windpipe

tracheostomy ____
____

trā kē os′ tō mē
a permanent opening into the windpipe

16.
Write the word root and combining form for windpipe:
__________________.

trache or trache/o

17.
A *bronchus* is one of the major divisions of the windpipe. The bronchi (plural) direct the air into the lungs. Write a meaning for each of the following:

bronchoscopy ____
____

brong kos′ kō pē
looking into the bronchus

bronchospasm ____
____

bron′ kō spazm
spasm of the bronchus

brong kī′ tis
inflammation of the bronchus or bronchi

bronchitis ______________________________

18.

bronch, bronch/o

The word root and combining form meaning major branches of the windpipe that open into the lungs is ______________.

19.

Pleural means pertaining to the covering on the lungs. The pleural membrane completely covers the lungs and clings to it like plastic wrap. Only a few drops of thick fluid keep the lung and the pleura apart.

plo͞o rī′ tis
inflammation of the pleura

Pleuritis means ______________________________.

pleuralgia or pleurodynia
plo͞o ral′ jē ə
plo͞o rō din′ ē ə

20.

Pleurisy is another word for inflammation of the covering of the lungs. Build a term that means pain in the pleura: ______________________________.

21.

plo͞o rō sen tē′ sis
puncture of the pleural space and removing the fluid

Pleurisy may cause excessive fluid to collect within the space between the lung and the pleura. A pleurocentesis can be used to diagnose pleurisy. What do you think pleurocentesis means? ______________________________

22.

diaphragm
dī′ a fram

Refer to Figure 11.1 again. The musculomembranous wall separating the abdomen from the chest cavity is the ______________.

23.

in

During inspiration the diaphragm contracts; it flattens out downward, permitting the lungs to move downward, or expand, and fill with air. Inspiration is breathing ______________ (in/out).

24.

out

During expiration the diaphragm relaxes. It resumes its inverted basin shape, squeezing the lungs and expelling the air out of the lungs. Expiration is breathing ______________ (in/out).

25.
The organ largely responsible for inspiration and expiration is the __________.

diaphragm

26.
A sudden spasm of the diaphragm usually produces a giggle all around. It is called singultus. Can you guess what it means? __________

hiccough, or hiccup
hik′ kof

27.
Another term for hiccough is __________.

singultus
sin gul′ tus

28.
Ptysis is a Greek term meaning spitting. What does hem/o/ptysis mean? __________

hē mop′ ti sis
spitting blood

29.
Hemoptysis means spitting blood (arising from hemorrhage of larynx, trachea, bronchi, or lungs). Write the suffix meaning spitting, or spitting up. __________

-ptysis (the p is silent)

What does hemat/emesis mean? __________

hē ma tem′ a sis
expelling blood from the stomach
(vomiting blood)

30.
Write the two combining forms for blood you just used in frames above. __________ and __________

hem/o, hemat/o

31.
Using either suffix, -ptysis or -emesis, build a medical term to express the following definitions:

spitting blood from hemorrhage of the lungs __________

hemoptysis

expelling blood from the stomach __________

hematemesis

32.
Epistaxis means nosebleed. What does rhinorrhagia mean? __________

rīn or ra′ jē a
hemorrhage from the nose

33.
Two terms mean bleeding from the nose. They are __________ and __________.

epistaxis
ep i stak′ sis
rhinorrhagia

Which term means severe bleeding from the nose? __________

rhinorrhagia

Answer	Frame
spitting blood (arising from the larynx, trachea, bronchi, or lungs)	34. What does hemoptysis mean? ________________________________
vomiting blood (from the stomach)	35. What does hematemesis mean? ________________________________
rhinorrhagia	36. Nasal hemorrhage is ________________ .
epistaxis	Nosebleed is ________________ .
nyōō mat′ ik pertaining to air or gases (or exchange of gases)	37. *Pneum/o, pneumat/o* mean air, gases, or exchange of gases. What does pneumatic mean? ________________________________
brad ip nē′ a breathing very slowly	38. Pne/o relates to breathing. Do you remember what bradypnea means? ________________________________
pne/o (nē ō)	39. The combining form referring to inhale and exhale, or in other words to breathe, is ____________________.
	Pneum/o, pneumat/o are combining forms meaning air, gases, or exchange of gases. Explain what these terms mean:
an abnormal condition of air in a joint	pneum/arthr/osis ________________________________
presence of air or gases in the blood of heart	pneumato/cardia ________________________________
air in the urine during or after urination	pneumat/uria ________________________________
pneum-	What is the word root for air or gases? ____________________
nyōō mol′ ō jē air or gases	40. Pneum/ology refers to the science of how the lungs exchange ____________________ or ____________________.
not breathing, breathing is absent	Apnea means ________________________________.

Answer	Frame
pneumotherapy nyo͞o mō ther′ ə pē	41. Hydrotherapy means treatment with water. Build a term meaning treatment with (compressed) air: ________________.
pneum/o pneumon/o	42. *Pneumon, pneumon/o* mean lung. At a quick glance you may confuse it with the root for air or gases. Write the combining forms for both: ________________ (air or gases); ________________ (lung).
pneumonitis nyo͞o mō nī′ tis pneumonectomy nyo͞o mōn ek′ tō mē	43. Pneumonia is a serious disease of the lung. Build a term for each of the following: inflammation of the lung ________________ surgical removal of a lung ________________
pne/o (nē ō)	44. Drawing air into the lungs and pushing air out of the lungs is called breathing. The combining form referring to breathing is ________________.
nyo͞o mon′ ō graf radiographic picture of the lungs (chest X ray)	45. Pneum/o/encephal/o/graphy means X ray examination of spaces within the brain. These X rays are taken following withdrawal of cerebrospinal fluid (via lumbar puncture) and replacement of it with injected air or gas. What is a pneumon/o/graph? ________________
breathing, breathe air or gas lung	46. Write a brief meaning for each of the following: pne/o ________________ pneum/o or pneumat/o ________________ pneumon/o ________________
thorax thor′ aks	47. *Thorax* encloses the chest cavity. It refers to the upper part of the trunk between the neck and the abdomen. The diaphragm separates the abdomen from the ________________.
thoracic cavity or thorax	48. The organs of the digestive apparatus are enclosed in the abdomen. The chief organs of the circulatory and respiratory systems are located in the ________________.

49.
Thorac and *thorac/o* are the word root and combining form referring to the chest cavity.

thor a cot′ ə mē
incision into the chest cavity

Thoracotomy means ______________________________ __________________.

thor a cō sen tē′ sis
puncture of the chest cavity to draw off fluid

Explain thoracocentesis: ______________________________ ______________________________

50.
Pneumothorax means air in the chest cavity. What does hemothorax mean? ______________________________

hē mō thor′ aks
blood in the chest cavity

51.
Let's conclude this unit with a review. Using the suggested answers, complete each of the following brief definitions. Write your answer in the space provided.

SUGGESTED ANSWERS:

bronchus(i)	pleura
diaphragm	trachea
larynx	singultus
pharynx	epistaxis

voice box ______________________________
main branches of the windpipe ______________________________
nosebleed ______________________________
windpipe ______________________________
hiccough ______________________________
throat ______________________________
tough film enveloping the lungs ______________________________
muscle controlling breathing ______________________________

larynx
bronchi
epistaxis
trachea
singultus
pharynx
pleura
diaphragm

52.
Try that again.

SUGGESTED ANSWERS:

apneic	hemoptysis
pneumothorax	rhinoplasty
pneumonogram	pneumonia
nasal	pleurodynia

pneumonia	serious lung condition ________
hemoptysis	spitting blood (arising from trachea) ________
pneumonogram	X ray of the lung(s) ________
pneumothorax	collection of air in the chest cavity ________
nasal	pertaining to the nose ________
rhinoplasty	a "nose job" ________
pleurodynia	pain in the pleura ________
apneic	pertaining to absence of breathing ________

53.

Here's one last exercise to show how far you have come! For each area of medical concern, write the term describing a practicing specialist

	AREA OF MEDICAL CONCERN	SPECIALIST
Pathologist	Bodily changes in structure and function due to disease	________
Psychiatrist	Mental illness	________
Dermatologist	Skin and its diseases	________
Gynecologist	Diseases of women	________
Cardiologist	Diseases of the heart	________
Neurologist	Nervous system diseases	________
Pediatrician	Childhood illnesses	________
Obstetrician	Pregnancy and childbirth	________
Ophthalmologist	Diseases of the eye	________
Urologist	Conditions of urogenitals	________

54.

Try it again. Describe the area of medical concern for these specialists.

	SPECIALIST	AREA OF MEDICAL CONCERN
Bones and muscles	Orthopedist	________
Pregnancy and childbirth	Obstetrician	________
Old age, aging	Geriatrician	________
Causes of epidemics	Epidemiologist	________
Skilled diagnosing	Diagnostician	________
Anesthesia and pain	Anesthesiologist	________
Urinary and genitals	Urologist	________
Tumors and treatment	Oncologist	________
Ear, nose, throat, and voice box	Otorhinopharyngo-laryngologist	________

55.

Here are 24 more medical terms you have worked with in Chapter 11. Don't forget to pronounce each one carefully before taking the final Chapter 11 Self-Test.

apnea (ap′ nē ə)
bradypnea (brad ip nē′ ə)
bronchitis (brong kī′ tis)
bronchoscopy (brong kos′ kō pē)
diaphragm (dī′ a fram)
epistaxis (ep i stak′ sis)
hemoptysis (hē mop′ ti sis)
laryngeal (la rin′ jē al)
laryngospasm (la ring′ gō spazm)
nasopharyngitis (nā′ zō fair in jī′ tis)
pharyngitis (fair in jī′ tis)
pharyngotomy (fair in got′ ō mē)
pleuralgia (plo͞o ral′ jē ə)
pleurisy (plo͞or′ i sē)
pleurocentesis (plo͞or′ ō sen tē′ sis)
pneumohemothorax (nyo͞o mō hē mō thōr′ aks)
pneumonia (nyo͞o mō′ nē ə)
rhinoplasty (ri′ nō plas tē)
singultus (sing gul′ tus)
tachypnea (tak ip nē′ ə)
tracheorrhagia (trā kē ō rāj′ jē ə)
tracheostomy (trā kē os′ tō mē)
thorax (thor′ aks)
thoracocentesis (thôr′ ə kō sen tē′ sis)

Chapter 11 Self-Test

Part 1

From the list on the right, select the correct meaning for each of the following often used medical terms.

______	1. Pneumonectomy	a.	Nosebleed
______	2. Pleurocentesis	b.	Spitting blood from the lungs
______	3. Pleuralgia	c.	Pertaining to nose and chin
______	4. Hemoptysis	d.	Puncture of the pleural space to remove fluid
______	5. Nasomental	e.	Pain of the pleura
______	6. Tracheorrhagia	f.	Hemorrhage from the trachea
______	7. Epistaxis	g.	Inflammation of the bronchi
______	8. Bronchitis	h.	Surgical removal of a lung
______	9. Bradypnea	i.	Abnormally slow breathing

Part 2

Write the medical term for each of the following brief definitions.

1. Air in the chest cavity ______________________
2. Incision into the throat ______________________
3. Hiccough ______________________
4. Pain in the covering of the lung ______________________
5. Permanent opening into the windpipe ______________________
6. Spasm of the voice box ______________________
7. Nosebleed ______________________
8. Very fast breathing ______________________

ANSWERS

Part 1

1. h
2. d
3. e
4. b
5. c
6. f
7. a
8. g
9. i

Part 2

1. Pneumothorax
2. Pharyngotomy
3. Singultus
4. Pleurodynia
5. Tracheostomy
6. Laryngospasm
7. Epistaxis
8. Tachypnea

Review by Body System Assessment

Medical professionals use a standard assessment order as they describe and check patients, which helps make sense of all the possible problems or normal findings for other practitioners that may follow the assessment. The following list contains the medical terminology you have learned in this book divided by body system. The list is not comprehensive, but it will give you a good idea of some of the most common terminology in each body system. It may help you to remember these groupings as you study. Remember the importance of this order as you review a client's chart or document your own findings. Consistency of terminology among medical professionals helps increase productivity and accuracy, and it is important to be as specific as possible.

Assessment by Body System

HEENT: head, eyes, ears, nose, and throat
Cardiac: heart, veins and arteries
Respiratory: lungs
Chest: shoulders to diaphragm, excluding heart and lungs
Abdomen: abdominal
GI: Gastrointestinal
GU: Genitourinary
Ext: Extremities

Medical Terminology by Body System

HEENT: Head, Eyes, Ears, Nose, and Throat

Adenitis: inflammation of a gland
Adenoma: tumor of a gland
Afebrile: without fever
Alopecia: absence of hair
Andontia: without teeth
Aphasia: speechless

Asymptomatic: without symptoms
Bradyphasia: abnormally slow speech
Cephalgia: head pain
Cephalalgia: headache
Cheilitis: inflammation of the lips
Cheilosis: abnormal condition of the lips
Corectopia: misplaced pupil
Cranioplasty: surgical repair of the skull
Craniotomy: incision into the skull
Cyclitis: inflammation of the cilliary body
Cyclokeratitis: inflammation of the cornea and the ciliary body
Dentalgia: tooth pain
Dysphasia: difficulty speaking
Encephalitis: inflammation of the brain
Encephalocele: herniation of the brain
Encephaloma: brain tumor
Gingivalgia: painful gums
Gingivectomy: excision of the gums
Gingivitis: inflammation of the gums
Gingivoglossitis: inflammation of the gums and tongue
Glossalgia: painful tongue
Glossectomy: excision of the tongue
Glossitis: inflammation of the tongue
Glossospasm: tongue spasm
Hydrocephalus: water on the head
Hyperpyrexia: fever over 106°F in an adult
Hyperthermic: body temperature above normal
Hyperthyroidism: excessive thyroid activity
Hypoglossal: under the tongue
Hypothermic: body temperature below normal
Iritis: inflammation of the iris
Keratopathy: disorder of the eye
Lacrimal gland: gland that secretes tears
Lacrimal sac: sac that collects tears
Laryngitis: inflammation of the voice box
Laryngospasm: spasm of the voice box
Macrocephalus: abnormally large head

Macrocheilia: abnormally large lips
Macroglossia: abnormally large tongue
Macrorhinia: abnormally large nose
Macrotia: abnormally large ears
Malaise: not feeling well
Myelocele: herniation of the spinal cord
Neuralgia: painful nerve
Neurofibroma: tumor containing nerve tissue
Neurosclerosis: hardening of a nerve tissue
Neurospasm: spasm of a nerve
Otalagia: ear pain
Otorrhea: discharge from the ear
Pyrexia: fever
Retina: complex membranous lining that receives the light rays in the eye
Retinitis: inflammation of the retina
Retinopathy: diease of the retina
Rhinitis: inflammation of the nose
Rhinorrhea: discharge from the nose
Stomatalgia: painful mouth
Stomatitis: inflammation of the mouth
Stomatorrhagia: hemorrhage of the mouth
Tachyphasia: abnormally fast speech
Tinnitus: ringing in the ears
Tracheotomy: temporary opening in the trachea
Vertigo: sensation of spinning

Cardiac: Heart, Veins, and Arteries

Angiorrhexis: rupture of a blood vessel
Angiosclerosis: hardening of a blood vessel
Angiospasm: spasm of a vessel
Arteriomalacia: softening of the arteries
Arteriosclerosis: hardening of the arteries
Arteriospasm: spasm of the arteries
Bradycardia: slow heartbeat
Cardiac arrest: cessation of heart function
Cardialgia: heart pain
Cardiomegaly: enlarged heart

Cardiorrhexis: rupture of the heart
Carditis: inflammation of the heart
Coronary thrombosis: blood clot in the coronary vessels
Defibrillation: utilizing an electrical impulse to restore a regular heartbeat
Electrocardiogram: record of electrical heart impulses
Endocarditis: inflammation of the inside of the heart
Embolism: sudden obstruction of a blood vessel
Embolus: foreign particle in circulation
Fibrillation: fast, irregular heartbeat
Phlebitis: inflammation of the vein
Phleborrhexis: rupture of a vein
Phleboscerosis: hardening of the veins
Phlebotomy: incision into the vein
Tachycardia: fast heartbeat
Thrombectomy: excision of a thrombus
Thrombosis: condition caused by a clot

Respiratory: Lungs

Apnea: without breathing
Bradypnea: slow breathing
Bronchitis: inflammation of the bronchus
Bronchospasm: spasm of the bronchus
Cheyne-Stokes: breathing pattern characterized by cyclical hyperpnea followed by apnea
Cyanosis: abnormal blue color
Dyspnea: difficult/painful breathing
Hemoptysis: hemorrhage of the lungs
Hemothorax: blood in the chest cavity
Hyperpnea: respirations > 25 r/min in an adult
Intercostal: space between the ribs
Paroxysmal dyspnea: sudden, recurring episode of difficult breathing
Pleurisy: pain in the pleura
Pleuritis: inflammation of the pleura
Pneumonitis: serious disease of the lung
Pneumothorax: air in the chest cavity
Singultus: hiccough

Tachypnea: fast breathing
Thoracocentesis: puncture of the thorax

Chest: Shoulders to Diaphragm, Excluding Heart and Lungs

Gynecomastia: abnormally large mammary glands in a male
Mastadenitis: inflammation of the mammary gland
Mastadenoma: tumor of the mammary gland
Mastectomy: surgical removal of the breast
Mastitis: inflammation of the breast
Mastocarcinoma: cancerous tumor of the mammary gland
Mastodynia: painful breast
Mastopathy: disease of the mammary gland
Mastoptosis: pendulous breasts
Thoracotomy: incision into the chest cavity

Abdomen: Abdominal

Abdominocentesis: abdominal fluid removal with a needle
Anorexia: loss of appetite
Cyanoderma: blue skin
Edema: accumulation of fluid in the body tissues
Erythroderma: red skin
Melanocarcinoma: black, malignant tumor
Melanoderma: black discolored skin
Orexia: appetite
Peritoneum: tough membrane covering the abdominal organs
Peritonitis: inflammation of the peritoneum

GI: Gastrointestinal

Cholecystectomy: surgical removal of the gallbladder
Cholecystitis: inflammation of the gallbladder
Cholemesis: bile in emesis
Coloclysis: irrigation of the colon
Colostomy: surgical opening into the colon
Duodenitis: inflammation of the duodenum
Dyspepsia: painful or poor digestion
Emesis: product of vomiting
Enterectasia: dilation of the small intestine

Enterocele: herniation of the small intestine
Enteroclysis: irrigation of the small intestine
Enterorrhexis: rupture of the small intestine
Esophagoduodenostomy: opening formed between the esophagus and duodenum
Gastralgia: stomach pain
Gastritis: inflammation of the stomach
Gastroectasia: dilation of the stomach
Gastroenteric: pertaining to the stomach and small intestine
Gastroenterostomy: surgical opening between the stomach and small intestine
Hematemesis: blood in emesis
Hepatitis: inflammation of the liver
Hepatomegaly: enlarged liver
Hepatorrhagia: hemorrhage of the liver
Hyperemesis: excessive vomiting
Megalogastria: enlarged stomach
Nausea: sensation or desire to vomit
Pancreatectomy: excision of all or part of the pancreas
Pancreatitis: inflammation of the pancreas
Pancreatolith: pancreatic stone
Proctolysis: irrigation of the rectum and anus
Rectocele: rectal hernia
Rectoclysis: irrigation of the rectum
Rectocolitis: inflammation of the rectum and colon

GU: Genitourinary

Amniocentesis: puncturing the amniotic sac and removing amniotic fluid
Amniotic fluid: liquid surrounding the fetus
Antepartum: period of time in pregnancy before labor begins
Colpitis: inflammation of the vagina
Colpospasm: vaginal spasm
Cryptorchidism: undecended testicles
Cystitis: inflammation of the bladder
Cystorrhagia: bladder hemorrhage
Cystorrhexis: rupture of the bladder
Cystotomy: temporary opening in the bladder

Ectopic: pregnancy outside the uterus
Embryo: complex organism eight weeks following conception
Fetus: product of conception from nine weeks to delivery
Gestation: pregnancy
Hysterectomy: surgical removal of the uterus
Hysteroptosis: sagging of the uterus
Hysterospasm: spasm of the uterus
Involution: uterus returning to its pre-pregnant size and shape
Metritis: inflammation of the uterine tissues
Metrorrhagia: uterine hemorrhage
Metrorrhea: mucous or pus discharge from the uterus
Nephroplasty: surgical repair of the kidney
Nulliparous: woman who has never been pregnant
Oligohydramnios: too little amniotic fluid
Oophorectomy: surgical removal of the ovary
Oophoritis: inflamed ovary
Oophoroma: ovarian tumor
Orchiditis: inflammation of the testicle
Orchidotomy: testicular incision
Ovum: female egg
Perineum: area between vaginal opening and anus in a female or scrotum and anus in a male
Polyhydramnios: too much amniotic fluid
Polyuria: excessive amounts of urine
Postpartum: period of time following the birth of a baby
Prenatal care: care given to a pregnant woman before childbirth
Primigravida: first pregnancy
Pudendum: female external sex organs
Pyelitis: inflammation of the renal pelvis
Pyelonephritis: inflammation of the renal pelvis and kidney
Salpingectomy: excision of the fallopian tube
Salpingitis: inflammation of the fallopian tube
Spermatozoon: male germ cell
Ureterolith: stone in the ureter
Ureterolithotomy: surgical removal of a stone in the ureter
Ureteropyelitis: inflammation of the ureter and renal pelvis
Urethrospasm: spasm of the urethra

Ext: Extremities

Acrocyanosis: abnormal blue color of the extremities
Acrodermatitis: inflammation of the extremity skin
Acromegaly: enlarged extremities
Arthritis: inflammation of the joints
Arthrotomy: temporary opening in a joint
Atrophy: underdevelopment of the tissues
Chondrodysplasia: defective development of cartilidge
Chondromalacia: softened cartilage
Cyanoderma: abnormal blue color of the skin
Dactylitis: inflammation of a digit
Dactylospasm: spasm of a digit
Dermatitis: inflammation of the skin
Dermatosis: abnormal skin condition
Hyperplasia: overdeveloped
Hypertrophy: overdeveloped tissues
Hypoplasia: underdeveloped
Kinesialgia: pain on movement
Luekoderm: abnormal white color of the skin
Macrodactylia: abnormally large fingers
Myofibroma: tumor containing muscle tissue
Myosclerosis: hardening of a muscle tissue
Myospasm: spasm of a muscle
Osteochondritis: inflammation of the bone and cartilage
Osteochondrodysplasia: defective formation of bone and cartilage
Peripheral: away from the center of the body
Polyarthritis: inflammation of many joints
Polydactylism: too many finger/toes
Polyneuralgia: pain in many nerves
Syndactylism: joining of one or more digits
Tendonitis: inflammation of the tendons

Review Sheets by Chapter

Chapter 1: Review Sheet

Part 1

Cover the column of words on the right. In the space provided write the meaning of each word part listed in the left column. Check your answers.

Word Part	Meaning	(Hide This Column)
acr/o-	____________	extremity
megal/o-	____________	enlargement
dermat/o-	____________	skin
cyan/o-	____________	blue
derm/o-	____________	skin
leuk/o-	____________	white
-itis	____________	inflammation
cardi/o-	____________	heart
gastr/o-	____________	stomach
cyt/o-	____________	cell
-ologist	____________	one who studies
-algia	____________	pain
-ectomy	____________	excision
-otomy	____________	incision
-ostomy	____________	new opening
duoden/o-	____________	duodenum
electr/o-	____________	electricity
-ology	____________	study of
-osis	____________	condition of
-tome	____________	instrument that cuts
gram/o-	____________	record
eti/o-	____________	cause of
path/o-	____________	disease

Part 2

Cover the word parts in the right-hand column. In the space provided write a suffix or word part that expresses the meaning of each word in the left column. Check your answers.

Meaning	Word Part	(Hide This Column)
record	____________	gram/o-
one who studies (suffix)	____________	-ologist
enlargement	____________	megal/o-
electric	____________	electr/o-
white	____________	leuk/o-
incision into (suffix)	____________	-otomy
blue	____________	cyan/o-
instrument that cuts (suffix)	____________	-tome
stomach	____________	gastr/o-
extremity	____________	acr/o-
(abnormal) condition of (suffix)	____________	-osis
changes due to disease	____________	path/o-
new opening formed (suffix)	____________	-ostomy
skin	____________	dermat/o-, dermat
study of (suffix)	____________	-ology
heart	____________	cardi/o-
excision (suffix)	____________	-ectomy
inflammation of (suffix)	____________	-itis
duodenum	____________	duoden/o-
pain (suffix)	____________	-algia
cell	____________	cyt/o-
cause of	____________	eti/o-

Chapter 2: Review Sheet

Part 1

Cover the column of words on the right. In the space provided write the meaning of the word parts listed in the left column. Check your answers.

Word Part	Meaning	(Hide This Column)
aden/o-	______	gland
carcin/o-	______	cancer
malac/o-	______	soft, softened
-oid	______	resembling
laryng/o-	______	larynx
cephal/o-	______	head
hyper-	______	excessive, more than normal
-cele	______	herniation
ost/o-, oste/o-	______	bone
arthr/o-	______	joint
chondr/o-	______	cartilage
cost/o-	______	rib
lip/o-	______	fat
inter-	______	between
dent/o-, dont/o	______	tooth
-emesis	______	vomiting
-oma	______	tumor
-plast/o, -plast/y	______	repair
hypo-	______	under, less than normal
troph/o-	______	development
morph/o-	______	structure and form
muc/o-	______	mucus
onc/o-	______	tumor
hist/o-	______	tissue(s)
en-, endo-	______	inside, within
ex-, exo-	______	out, completely outside

Part 2

Cover the column on the right while you work. In the space provided, write the word part or combining form that matches the definition listed in the left column.

Meaning	Word Part	(Hide This Column)
rib	______________	cost/o-
larynx	______________	laryng/o-
development	______________	troph/o-
cancer	______________	carcin/o-
repair (suffix)	______________	-plast/o(/y)
tooth	______________	dent/o-, dont/o
mucus	______________	muc/o-
under, less than normal	______________	hypo-
herniation (suffix)	______________	-cele
soft, softened	______________	malac/o-
gland	______________	aden/o-
tumor (suffix)	______________	-oma
bone	______________	oste/o-
vomiting (suffix)	______________	-emesis
head	______________	cephal/o-
joint	______________	arthr/o-
between (prefix)	______________	inter-
resembling (suffix)	______________	-oid
fat	______________	lip/o-
inside, within (prefix)	______________	en-, endo-
cartilage	______________	chondr/o-
excessive, more than normal (prefix)	______________	hyper-
tissue	______________	hist/o-
structure and form	______________	morph/o-
tumor(s)	______________	onc/o-
out, completely outside (prefix)	______________	ex-, exo-

Chapter 3: Review Sheet

Part 1

Cover the column of words on the right. In the space provided write the meaning of each word part listed in the left column. Check your answers.

Word Part	Meaning	(Hide This Column)
cyst/o-	________________	bladder
-ar	________________	pertaining to
crani/o-	________________	cranium (skull)
dipl/o-	________________	double
ab-	________________	away from
cocc/i-	________________	coccus
metr/o, meter-	________________	measure
py/o-	________________	pus
-genesis, gen/o-	________________	produce, originate
-orrhea	________________	flow
ot/o-	________________	ear
-centesis	________________	puncture
rhin/o-	________________	nose
lith/o-	________________	stone or calculus
hydro-	________________	water
chol/e-	________________	gall, bile
thorac/o-	________________	thorax or chest
pelv/i-	________________	pelvis
ad-	________________	toward
abdomin/o-	________________	abdomen
therap/o-	________________	treatment
cephal/o-	________________	head, cranium
phob/ia	________________	fear
cardi/o	________________	heart

Part 2

Cover the word parts on the right. In the space provided write a term that expresses the meaning of each word in the left column. Check your answers.

Meaning	Word Part	(Hide This Column)
water, watery fluid	______	hydro-
flow, discharge (suffix)	______	-orrhea
abnormal fear	______	phob/ia
double, pairs	______	dipl/o-
head	______	cephal/o
pelvis	______	pelv/i-
gall, bile	______	chol/e-
nose	______	rhin/o-
puncture of a cavity (suffix)	______	-centesis
pus	______	py/o-
treatment	______	therap/o-
toward the midline (prefix)	______	ad-
produce, originate (suffix, prefix)	______	-genesis, gen/o-
bladder	______	cyst/o-
coccus	______	cocc/i-, cocc/o
measure	______	metr/o-, meter-
stone or calculus	______	lith/o-
ear	______	ot/o-
thorax or chest	______	thorac/o-
cranium (skull)	______	crani/o-
away from the midline (prefix)	______	ab-
abdomen	______	abdomin/o-

Chapter 4: Review Sheet

Part 1

Cover the right-hand column. Write the meaning of each word or word part in the left column. Be sure to check your answers.

Word/ Word Part	Meaning	(Hide This Column)
-peps/ia	__________	digestion
neur/o-	__________	nerve
blast/o-	__________	immature cell form, germ cell
a-, an-	__________	without
angi/o-	__________	vessel
-spasm	__________	twitching, spasm
scler/o-	__________	hard, hardened
aneurysm	__________	ballooning-out vessel
fibr/o-	__________	fibrous, fiber
lys/o-	__________	destruction, dissolution
arteri/o-	__________	artery
men/o-	__________	menses, menstruation
hemat/o-, hemo-	__________	blood
kinesi/o-	__________	movement
spermat/o-	__________	spermatozoon, spermatozoa (plural)
oophor/o-	__________	ovary
-pexy	__________	fixation
salping/o-	__________	fallopian tube
dys-	__________	bad, painful, difficult
hyster/o-	__________	uterus
-ptosis	__________	prolapse, drooping
anomaly	__________	irregularity, breaks the rule
ur/o-	__________	urine
nephr/o-	__________	kidney
pyel/o-	__________	renal pelvis
ureter/o-	__________	ureter

(continued on next page)

-orrhaphy	______________	to suture, repair
urethr/o-	______________	urethra
-orrhagia	______________	hemorrhage
colp/o-	______________	vagina
crypt/o-	______________	hidden
orchid/o-	______________	testis, testes (plural)
hernia	______________	protrusion through cavity wall

Part 2

Cover the word parts on the right. In the space provided write a term that expresses the meaning of each word in the left column. Check your answers.

Meaning	Word/Word Part	(Hide This Column)
artery	______________	arteri/o-
vessel	______________	angi/o-
uterus	______________	hyster/o-
movement	______________	kinesi/o-
destruction, dissolution	______________	lys/o-
blood	______________	hemat/o-, hem/o-
protrusion through cavity wall	______________	hernia
urine	______________	ur/o-
hard, hardening	______________	scler/o-
fallopian tube	______________	salping/o-
muscle	______________	my/o-
without (prefix)	______________	a-, an-
nerve	______________	neur/o-
surgical fixation (suffix)	______________	-pexy
germ cell (immature)	______________	blast/o-
ballooning-out vessel	______________	aneurysm
ovary	______________	oophor/o-
digestion	______________	-peps/ia
prolapse, drooping	______________	-ptosis
bad, painful, difficult (prefix)	______________	dys-
spermatozoa (pl.)	______________	spermat/o-
fibrous, fiber	______________	fibr/o-
twitching (suffix)	______________	-spasm
fast, rapid (prefix)	______________	tachy-
hemorrhage (suffix)	______________	-orrhagia
renal pelvis	______________	pyel/o-
vagina	______________	colp/o-
ureter	______________	ureter/o-
kidney	______________	nephr/o-

(continued on next page)

irregularity, breaks the rule	______________	anomaly
urethra	______________	urethr/o-
to suture, repair (suffix)	______________	-orrhaphy
hidden	______________	crypt/o-
testes (pl.)	______________	orchid/o-
menses, menstruation	______________	men/o-

Congratulations!

Chapter 5: Review Sheet

Part 1

Cover the right-hand column. Write the meaning of each word or word part in the left column. Be sure to check your answers.

Word/ Word Part	Meaning	(Hide This Column)
stomat/o-	______	mouth
gloss/o-	______	tongue
cheil/o-	______	lips
gingiv/o-	______	gums
esophag/o-	______	esophagus
enter/o-	______	small intestine
-scope	______	instrument to look, examine
col/o-	______	colon
rect/o-	______	rectum
proct/o-	______	anus and rectum
hepat/o-	______	liver
pancreat/o-	______	pancreas
clys/o, -clysis	______	wash, irrigate
-ectasia	______	dilation, stretching
-spasm	______	twitching, cramping
dent/o-	______	teeth, tooth
toxin	______	poison, poisoning
hypo-	______	under, beneath
hyper-	______	excessive
-algia	______	pain, ache
-osis	______	abnormal, diseased condition
-ostomy	______	surgery to form a new opening (permanent)
-otomy	______	incision into
-ectomy	______	surgical removal of
-pexy	______	surgical fixation of a part in its normal place

Part 2

Cover the word parts on the right. In the space provided write a term that expresses the meaning of each word in the left column. Check your answers.

Meaning	Word/Word Part	(Hide This Column)
cramping, twitching	______________	spasm
liver	______________	hepat/o-
excessive (prefix)	______________	hyper-
small intestine	______________	enter/o-
surgical incision into (suffix)	______________	-otomy
surgery to form a new opening (suffix)	______________	-ostomy
pertaining to teeth	______________	dental
rectum and anus	______________	proct/o-
lips	______________	cheil/o-
wash, irrigate (suffix)	______________	-clysis
esophagus	______________	esophag/o-
colon	______________	col/o-
gums	______________	gingiv/o-
mouth	______________	stomat/o-
pain, ache (suffix)	______________	-algia
dilation, stretching (a suffix)	______________	-ectasia
pancreas	______________	pancreat/o-
rectum	______________	rect/o-
tongue	______________	gloss/o-
surgical fixation of a part in normal place (suffix)	______________	-pexy
look, examine (suffix)	______________	-scopy

Chapter 6: Review Sheet

Part 1

Cover the right-hand column. Write the meaning of each word or word part listed in the left-hand column in the space provided. Be sure to check your answers.

Word/ Word Part	Meaning	(Hide This Column)
phleb/o-	____________	vein
dys-	____________	bad, difficult, painful
-orrhexis	____________	rupture, bursting apart
-esthesia	____________	sensation, feeling
fibrillation	____________	very rapid heartbeat
-algesia	____________	sensation of pain
phas/o-	____________	speech
thrombosis	____________	occlusion of a blood vessel by a blood clot
-tripsy	____________	surgical crushing
plas/o-	____________	formation, development
syn-, sym	____________	together as one
a-, an-	____________	without, absent
embolus	____________	foreign particle floating in blood-stream
dactyl/o-	____________	fingers, toes, digits
cardiac arrest	____________	cessation of heartbeat
-emia	____________	blood
embolism	____________	vessel occluded, blocked by an em-bolus
myel/o-	____________	spinal cord or bone marrow
poly-	____________	many
micro-	____________	very small, microscopic
defibrillation	____________	restoration of regular heartbeat (often with electric shock)
thrombus	____________	blood clot in the bloodstream

Part 2

Cover the word parts on the right. In the space provided write a term that expresses the meaning of each word in the left column. Check your answers.

Meaning	Word/Word Part	(Hide This Column)
a blood clot in the bloodstream	______________	thrombus
sensation, feeling	______________	-esthesia
speech	______________	phas/o-
sensation of pain	______________	-algesia
vein	______________	phleb/o-
vessel occluded by an embolus	______________	embolism
restoration of regular heartbeat, often by electric shock	______________	defibrillation
foreign particle circulating in the bloodstream	______________	embolus
formation, development in the sense of shaping, molding	______________	plas/o-
rupture, bursting apart (suffix)	______________	-orrhexis
bad, difficult, painful (prefix)	______________	dys-
surgical crushing (suffix)	______________	-tripsy
very, very small (prefix)	______________	micro-
large, seen by human eye (prefix)	______________	macro-
bone marrow or spinal cord	______________	myel/o-
finger or toe, digit	______________	dactyl/o-
many (prefix)	______________	poly-
together as one (prefix)	______________	syn-, sym-
very fast heartbeat	______________	fibrillation
blood (suffix)	______________	-emia

Chapter 7: Review Sheet

Part 1

Cover the right-hand column. Write the meaning of each word or word part listed in the left-hand column in the space provided. Be sure to check your answers.

Word/ Word Part	Meaning	(Hide This Column)
edema	______________	fluid in the tissues
chronic	______________	long, drawn-out disease
syndrome	______________	symptoms occur together
prognosis	______________	prediction of course and outcome of disease
acute	______________	pertaining to severe symptom, rapid onset, short course
paroxysmal	______________	pertaining to sudden periodic attack
diagnosis	______________	identification of disease
tinnitus	______________	ringing in the ear
malaise	______________	vague sensation of not feeling well
vertigo	______________	sensation of turning around in space
anorexia	______________	loss of appetite
symptom	______________	perceived change in body or functions
pyrexia	______________	feverishness
mortality	______________	pertaining to being mortal
morbidity	______________	pertaining to being diseased
hypertrophy	______________	overdevelopment
atrophy	______________	wasting away, shrinking of an organ

(continued on next page)

systemic ______	pertaining to the whole body, all systems
vital signs ______	T, P, and R
peripheral ______	pertaining to the outside surface of the body
chlor/o- ______	green
melan/o- ______	black
erythr/o- ______	red
xanth/o- ______	yellow
prophylactic ______	pertaining to prevention of disease
prodromal ______	pertaining to phase of disease before symptoms
nausea ______	seasickness, inclined to vomit
palliative ______	pertaining to relief of symptoms, not cure
against (prefix) ______	anti-
dyspnea ______	difficult, painful breathing
hypothermia ______	subnormal temperature, below 90°F

Part 2

Cover the word parts on the right. In the space provided write a term that expresses the meaning of each word in the left column. Check your answers.

Meaning	Word Part	(Hide This Column)
symptoms and signs occur together	____________	syndrome
prediction of course and outcome of disease	____________	prognosis
pertaining to severe symptom, rapid onset, short course	____________	acute
wasting away, shrinking of an organ	____________	atrophy
pertaining to the whole body, all systems	____________	systemic
T, P, and R	____________	vital signs
fluid in the tissues	____________	edema
long, drawn-out disease	____________	chronic
pertaining to sudden periodic attack	____________	paroxysmal
identification of disease	____________	diagnosis
ringing in the ear	____________	tinnitus
vague sensation of not feeling well	____________	malaise
sensation of turning around in space	____________	vertigo
loss of appetite	____________	anorexia
perceived change in body or functions	____________	symptom
statistic pertaining to being diseased	____________	morbidity

(continued on next page)

pertaining to relief of symptoms, not cure	________________	palliative
fever	________________	pyret/o-, pyrexia
pertaining to phase of disease before symptoms	________________	prodromal
pertaining to prevention of disease	________________	prophylactic
yellow	________________	xanth/o-
red	________________	erythr/o-
seasickness, inclined to vomit	________________	nausea
black	________________	melan/o-
green	________________	chlor/o-
pertaining to the outside surface of the body	________________	peripheral
breathing reaches a climax, then ceases before starting again	________________	Cheyne-Stokes respiration
difficult, painful breathing	________________	dyspnea
overdevelopment	________________	hypertrophy
statistic pertaining to being mortal	________________	mortality
feverishness	________________	pyret/o-, pyrexia
loss of appetite	________________	anorexia
symptoms occurring before the onset of the disease	________________	prodrome

Chapter 8: Review Sheet

Part 1

Cover the right-hand column. Write the meaning of each word or word part listed in the left-hand column in the space provided. Be sure to check your answers.

Word/ Word Part	Meaning	(Hide This Column)
supra-, super-	______	above, over
cyst	______	closed sac containing fluid
neoplasm	______	new tissue growth, no purpose
lesion	______	unhealthy, diseased tissue
infra-	______	below, beneath, under
ectopic	______	outside the normal place
ect/o-	______	outside
papule, papula	______	raised red spot, pimple
peri-, circum-	______	around, about, nearby
ventral	______	on or near the belly
epi-	______	over, upon, surrounding
distal	______	point farthest from trunk
dorsal	______	on or near the back
epigastric	______	area of the belly over the stomach
proximal	______	point nearest to the trunk
papilloma	______	nipple-shaped tumor on skin
lateral	______	farther from the midline
infiltration	______	slipping into and between normal cells

(continued on next page)

sub-, hypo-	______________	below, beneath
excrescence	______________	outgrowth, wart
medial	______________	nearer to the midline
papilla	______________	small, nipple-like protuberance
condyloma	______________	perianal wartlike growth
benign	______________	not spreading, not malignant
end/o-	______________	inner, inside
malignant	______________	bad kind, threatening death
tumor, neoplasm	______________	new, abnormal tissue growth
metastasis	______________	cells spread to new location
polyp	______________	tumor on a little foot, or stem
circumscribed	______________	as a line drawn around, edge
mes/o-	______________	middle

Part 2

Cover the word parts on the right. In the space provided write a term that expresses the meaning of each word in the left column. Check your answers.

Meaning	Word Part	(Hide This Column)
new, abnormal tissue growth	______________	tumor
cells spread to new location	______________	metastasis
middle (prefix)	______________	mes/o-
point nearest to the trunk	______________	proximal
perianal wartlike growth	______________	condyloma
not spreading, not malignant	______________	benign
inner, inside (prefix)	______________	end/o-
bad kind, threatening death	______________	malignant
closed sac containing fluid	______________	cyst
as a line drawn around, edge	______________	circumscribed
area of the belly over the stomach	______________	epigastric
new tissue growth, no purpose	______________	neoplasm
unhealthy, diseased tissue	______________	lesion
beneath the patella	______________	subpatellar, infrapatellar
outside the normal place	______________	ectopic
raised red spot, pimple	______________	papule, papula
around, circular (prefix)	______________	circum-
on or near the belly	______________	ventral

(continued on next page)

above the pubic arch	______________	suprapubic
below, beneath, under (prefix)	______________	infra-, sub-, hypo-
on or near the back	______________	dorsal
slipping into and between normal cells	______________	infiltration
tumor on a little foot	______________	polyp
over, surrounding (prefix)	______________	epi-
around, about, nearby (prefix)	______________	peri-
under the skin	______________	hypodermic
point farthest from trunk	______________	distal
nipple-shaped tumor on skin	______________	papilloma
farther from the midline	______________	lateral
removal and examination of living tissue	______________	biopsy

Chapter 9: Review Sheet

Part 1

Cover the right-hand column. Write the meaning of each word or word part listed in the left-hand column in the space provided. Be sure to check your answers.

Word/ Word Part	Meaning	(Hide This Column)
conception	__________	union of ovum and spermatozoon
ovum	__________	female egg cell
peritoneum	__________	thin membrane that coats the viscera and lines the abdominal wall
secundi-	__________	second
fetus	__________	developing child in utero
spermatozoon	__________	male germ cell
parturition	__________	labor and delivery of term pregnancy
multi-	__________	many
nulli-	__________	none
postpartum	__________	time period after giving birth
mastopathy	__________	breast disease
hysterorrhexis	__________	rupture of uterus (life-threatening)
metratrophy	__________	uterine atrophy
antepartum	__________	time period before labor
prenatal	__________	before childbirth
oligo-hydramnios	__________	scanty amount of amniotic fluid
mamm/o-, mast/o-	__________	breast
amniot/o-	__________	amnion (sac for fetus and fluid)
-atrophy	__________	wasting of an organ or part

(continued on next page)

primipara	______________________________	a woman who has given birth for the first time
-dynia	______________________________	pain, painful
-mania	______________________________	madness
-phobia	______________________________	excessive fear
-gravida	______________________________	heavy with child; a pregnant woman
men/o-	______________________________	menses, menstruation
involution	______________________________	process of uterus returning to nonpregnant state
climacteric	______________________________	change of life period
placenta	______________________________	organ that nourishes fetus in utero
gynecomastia	______________________________	enlarged breasts in a male
puerperium	______________________________	period after childbirth; involution takes place
pudenda	______________________________	female external genitals
gestation	______________________________	another term for pregnancy
amniocentesis	______________________________	puncture of amniotic sac and removal of fluid
perineum	______________________________	pelvic floor; region from vaginal lip to anus in female

Part 2

Cover the word parts on the right. In the space provided write a term that expresses the meaning of each word in the left column. Check your answers.

Meaning	Word Part	(Hide This Column)
female external genitals	______	pudenda
menses, menstruation	______	men/o-
madness (suffix)	______	-mania
female egg cell	______	ovum
wasting of an organ or part (suffix)	______	-atrophy
another term for pregnancy	______	gestation
puncture of amniotic sac and removal of fluid	______	amniocentesis
enlarged breasts in a male	______	gynecomastia
breast disease	______	mastopathy
breast (2 combining forms)	______	mast/o-, mamm/o-
none (prefix)	______	nulli-
many (prefix)	______	multi-
developing child in utero	______	fetus
male germ cell	______	spermatozoon
cessation of menses	______	menopause
pregnant woman, first time	______	primigravida
incision of vagina and pelvic outlet	______	episiotomy
excessive fear (prefix)	______	phobia-
pain, painful (suffix)	______	-dynia, -algia
process of uterus returning to nonpregnant state	______	involution
rupture of uterus (life-threatening)	______	hysterorrhexis

(continued on next page)

woman who has given birth to a living child	______________	para
pelvic floor; region from vaginal lip to anus in female	______________	perineum
period after childbirth; involution takes place	______________	puerperium
amnion (sac for fetus and fluid)	______________	amni/o-, amniot/o-
organ that nourishes fetus in utero	______________	placenta
few, little, scanty (prefix)	______________	oligo-
before labor	______________	antepartum
change-of-life period	______________	climacteric
physician specialist in diseases of women	______________	gynecologist
before (prefix)	______________	pre-
after (prefix)	______________	post-
new, recent (prefix)	______________	neo-
labor and delivery of term pregnancy	______________	parturition
X ray examination of breast	______________	mammography
thin membrane that coats viscera and abdominal wall	______________	peritoneum
union of ovum and spermatozoon	______________	conception
uterine atrophy	______________	metratrophy
pain, painful (suffix)	______________	-dynia, -algia
heavy with child; a pregnant woman	______________	gravida

Chapter 10: Review Sheet

Part 1

Cover the right-hand column. Write the meaning of each word or word part listed in the left-hand column in the space provided. Be sure to check your answers.

Word/ Word Part	Meaning	(Hide This Column)
scler/o-	______________	hard white coat of the eye
ir, irid/o-	______________	iris, donut-shaped color of the eye
dipl/o-	______________	double, paired
ophthalm/o-	______________	eye
retin/o-	______________	retina, complex membrane on the inside back surface of the eyeball
core-, core/o-	______________	pupil, circular opening in the center of the eye
lacrim/o-	______________	tear, tears
kerat/o-, corne/o-	______________	cornea, transparent covering of anterior one-sixth of the eye
-opia	______________	suffix meaning vision
cycl/o-	______________ ______________	ciliary body, controls the shape of the iris

Part 2

Cover the word parts on the right. In the space provided write a term that expresses the meaning of each word in the left column. Check your answers.

Meaning	Word Part	(Hide This Column)
iris	__________	ir-, irid/o-
cornea, transparent anterior covering of one-sixth of the eye	__________	kerat/o-, corne/o-
suffix meaning vision	__________	-opia
retina, complex membrane on the inside back surface of the eyeball	__________	retin/o-
eyelid	__________	blephar/o-
tear, tears	__________	lacrim/o-
pupil, circular opening in the center of the eye	__________	cor-, core-, core/o-
ciliary body, controls shape of the iris	__________	cycl/o-
hard white coat of the eye	__________	scler/o-
double, paired	__________	dipl/o-
eye	__________	ophthalm/o-

Chapter 11: Review Sheet

Part 1

Cover the right-hand column. Write the meaning of each word or word part listed in the left-hand column in the space provided. Be sure to check your answers.

Word/ Word Part	Meaning	(Hide This Column)
nas/o-	______	nose
pharyng/o-	______	pharynx, throat
laryng/o-	______	larynx, voice box
pneumon/o-	______	lung
bronch/o-	______	bronchus(i), branches of the trachea
pleur/o-	______	pleura, covering on the lungs
pne/o-	______	breathing, breathe
ment/o-	______	chin
thorac/o-	______	thorax, chest
pneum/o-	______	air, gases
trache/o-	______	windpipe, trachea
singultus	______	hiccup, hiccough
hemoptysis	______	spitting of blood derived from the lungs, bronchi
diaphragm	______	musculo-membranous wall separating the abdomen from the thorax
epistaxis	______	nosebleed

Part 2

Cover the word parts on the right. In the space provided write a term that expresses the meaning of each word in the left column. Check your answers.

Meaning	Word Part	(Hide This Column)
nose	______________	nas/o-
breathing, breathe	______________	pne/o-
larynx, voice box	______________	laryng/o-
nosebleed	______________	epistaxis
spitting blood derived from the lungs, trachea	______________	hemoptysis
musculomembranous wall separating the abdomen from the thorax	______________	diaphragm
air, gases	______________	pneum/o-
pleura, covering on the lungs	______________	pleur/o-
windpipe, trachea	______________	trache/o-
pharynx, throat	______________	pharyng/o-
bronchus(i), branches of the trachea	______________	bronch/o-
lung	______________	pneumon/o-
thorax, chest	______________	thorac/o-
chin	______________	ment/o-
hiccup, hiccough	______________	singultus

Congratulations on finishing your lessons.

Take the Final Tests after some rest and relaxation.

Final Self-Test I

Instructions

The following two tests will show you how much you have learned about medical terminology. Many of the words on the tests will be new to you; however, using the word parts and the word-building system you have learned, you should be able to give the meaning for all of them. Try these tests and see how well you do. You may want to take one test before reading the book and the other after you finish the book. The comparison will show even more clearly how much medical terminology you have learned.

Each test consists of 50 medical terms. For each term, write out a definition in your own words. Then compare your answers with those following the test. Your definition should include all of the ideas (though not necessarily in the exact words) as the definitions on the answer page.

1. Tachypnea ______________________
2. Oophoritis ______________________
3. Pyelonephrosis ______________________
4. Pathogenic ______________________
5. Bradycardia ______________________
6. Cycloparalysis ______________________
7. Glossoplegia ______________________
8. Megalodontia ______________________
9. Ophthalmoscopy ______________________
10. Bronchopneumonogram ______________________
11. Mammopexy ______________________
12. Cystocele ______________________
13. Cephalometer ______________________
14. Herniorrhaphy ______________________
15. Hyperthyroidism ______________________
16. Bronchiectasis ______________________

17. Mastodynia ______
18. Xanthemia ______
19. Symptomatology ______
20. Etiology ______
21. Kinesialgia ______
22. Fibroosteoma ______
23. Anuria ______
24. Lipochondroma ______
25. Costectomy ______
26. Ureteroenterostomy ______
27. Metrorrhagia ______
28. Paranephritis ______
29. Blepharoptosis ______
30. Erythrocyte ______
31. Perianal ______
32. Endocarditis ______
33. Lymphadenoid ______
34. Thoracolumbar ______
35. Corneoiritis ______
36. Hysterorrhexis ______
37. Thrombogenesis ______
38. Hematemesis ______
39. Lithotripsy ______
40. Oligohydramnios ______
41. Prostatic hypertrophy ______
42. Hemoptysis ______
43. Dorsalgia ______
44. Endocranial ______
45. Parturition ______
46. Adenocarcinoma ______
47. Esophagogastrostomy ______
48. Enterohepatitis ______
49. Malaise ______
50. Dyspnea ______

Answers to Final Self-Test I

1. rapid breathing
2. inflammation of an ovary
3. condition (abnormal or diseased) of the pelvis of the kidney
4. that which is capable of causing disease
5. slow heart rate
6. paralysis of the ciliary body
7. paralysis of the tongue
8. excessively large teeth
9. examination of the interior of the eye
10. X ray of the bronchi and lungs
11. surgical fixation of a breast to its normal position
12. hernia of the bladder
13. instrument for measuring the head
14. suturing (repair) of a hernia
15. condition caused by excessive secretion of the thyroid glands
16. dilatation of the bronchi
17. painful breast
18. yellow pigment (color) in the blood
19. the study (science) of disease symptoms
20. the study of causes of disease
21. painful muscular movement
22. tumor of bone and fibrous connective tissue
23. absence of urine
24. tumor of cartilaginous and fatty tissue
25. excision of a rib or ribs
26. make a permanent opening between the ureter and intestine
27. uterine hemorrhage
28. inflammation of tissues around (surrounding) the kidney
29. drooping of an eyelid
30. red blood cell
31. of or pertaining to around the anus
32. inflammation of the inside (lining) of the heart
33. resembling a lymph gland
34. of or pertaining to the chest (thorax) and lower back (lumbar)
35. inflammation of the iris and cornea
36. rupture of the uterus
37. formation (development) of a clot (thrombus)
38. vomiting blood
39. crushing removal of a stone
40. scanty amniotic fluid
41. pertaining to enlargement of the prostate
42. spitting blood (from trachea, bronchi, or lungs)
43. pain in the back
44. of, or pertaining to, the inside of the head
45. labor and childbirth
46. malignant tumor of a gland
47. making a new opening (permanent) between the esophagus and the stomach
48. inflammation of the liver and intestine
49. vague sensation of not feeling well
50. difficult or painful breathing

Final Self-Test II

1. Mastoptosis ______________________________
2. Epistaxis ______________________________
3. Amenorrhea ______________________________
4. Antipyretic ______________________________
5. Nephrolith ______________________________
6. Enterectasia ______________________________
7. Paroxysmal ______________________________
8. Encephalorrhagia ______________________________
9. Craniocele ______________________________
10. Anorexia ______________________________
11. Gingivoglossitis ______________________________
12. Cholecystitis ______________________________
13. Abdominalgia ______________________________
14. Arteriospasm ______________________________
15. Adenosclerosis ______________________________
16. Duodenohepatic ______________________________
17. Endobronchoscopy ______________________________
18. Iridoplegia ______________________________
19. Tracheostomy ______________________________
20. Syndactyly ______________________________
21. Phleborrhexis ______________________________
22. Cryptorchidism ______________________________
23. Thromboid ______________________________
24. Electroencephalogram ______________________________
25. Myelodysplasia ______________________________
26. Singultus ______________________________

27. Intercostal ______________________________
28. Epigastric ______________________________
29. Urethrocystitis ______________________________
30. Hypothyroidism ______________________________
31. Traumatology ______________________________
32. Pericardiectomy ______________________________
33. Syndrome ______________________________
34. Hepatorrhaphy ______________________________
35. Megalodactylism ______________________________
36. Nephropexy ______________________________
37. Pneumonomelanosis ______________________________
38. Cerebrovascular ______________________________
39. Chondromalacia ______________________________
40. Amniocentesis ______________________________
41. Inframammary ______________________________
42. Leukocytolysis ______________________________
43. Salpingectomy ______________________________
44. Hemodialysis ______________________________
45. Metastasis ______________________________
46. Cyanopia ______________________________
47. Ophthalmopathy ______________________________
48. Pneumohemothorax ______________________________
49. Otorhinolaryngologist ______________________________
50. Primagravida ______________________________

Answers to Final Self-Test II

1. pendulous, drooping breast
2. nosebleed
3. cessation of menstruation
4. a substance that counteracts (acts against) the effects of a fever
5. a stone (calculus) in the kidney
6. dilatation (stretching) of the small intestine
7. of, or pertaining to, a sudden recurrent onset of a condition (convulsions)
8. hemorrhage within the brain
9. hernia of structures in the skull (cranium)
10. loss of appetite
11. inflammation of the gums and tongue
12. inflammation of the gallbladder
13. painful abdomen
14. spasm (twitching) of an artery
15. condition of hardening of glandular tissue
16. of, or pertaining to, the duodenum and liver
17. examination of the inside of the bronchi
18. paralysis of the iris
19. making a new permanent opening in the trachea
20. webbing or fusion of fingers or toes
21. rupture of a vein
22. condition due to hidden (undescended) testes
23. resembling a blood clot
24. record (picture) of electrical activity in the brain
25. abnormal development of the spinal cord
26. hiccup, hiccough
27. between the ribs
28. of, or pertaining to, area of belly over stomach
29. inflammation of the urethra and bladder
30. condition of insufficient thyroid excretion
31. the study (science) of injuries and their effect on the body
32. excision of tissue around the heart
33. a group of symptoms occurring together
34. suturing (repairing) the liver
35. condition of abnormally large fingers and toes
36. surgical fixation of the kidney in its normal place
37. condition of black lungs, black lung disease
38. of, or pertaining to, the vessels of the brain
39. condition of softened cartilage tissue
40. puncture of the amniotic sac and withdrawing of fluid
41. below the breast
42. destruction of white blood cells
43. surgical removal of the fallopian tube
44. removal of toxic waste products from the blood
45. spreading of a malignant disease to another organ or location
46. blue vision
47. abnormal condition of the eyes
48. air and blood in the chest cavity
49. physician specialist in ear, nose, and voice box diseases
50. a woman pregnant for the first time

Appendix A Medical Abbreviations

$\bar{a}$	before
ad lib.	freely as desired (*ad libitum*)
ADL	activities of daily living
AMA	against medical advice
BBT	basal body temperature
bid; b.i.d.	twice a day (*bis in die*)
BM	bowel movement
BMR	basal metabolic rate
BP	blood pressure
bpm	beats per minute
BRP	bathroom privileges
BSE	breast self-examination
BUN	blood urea nitrogen
Bx	biopsy
C	carbon; Celsius
$\bar{c}$	with
Ca	calcium; cancer
CABG	coronary artery bypass graft
CAD	coronary artery disease
cath	catheter
CBC	complete blood count
CHD	congenital heart disease; coronary heart disease
CHF	congestive heart failure
CNS	central nervous system
c/o	complaints of
CO_2	carbon dixoxide
COPD	chronic obstructive pulmonary disease

CP	cerebral palsy; cleft palate
CPR	cardiopulmonary resuscitation
CT	computed tomography
CV	cardiovascular; closing volume
CVA	cerebrovasular accident; costovertebral angle
CXR	chest x-ray
DIC	disseminated intravascular coagulation
DKA	diabetes ketoacidosis
DM	diabetes mellitus, diastolic murmur
DNA	deoxyribonucleic acid
DNR	do not resuscitate
dr	dram
DTR	deep tendon reflex
D5W	dextrose 5% in water
Dx	diagnosis
ECG; EKG	electrocardiogram, electrocardiograph
ECHO	echocardiography
EEG	electroencephalogram, electroencephalograph
EENT	eye, ear, nose & throat
EOM	extraocular movement
FBS	fasting blood sugar
Fe	iron
Fl, fld	fluid
fl dr	fluid dram
fl oz	fluid ounce
fx	fracture
Gm; g; gm	gram
GFR	glomerular filtration rate
GI	gastrointestinal
gr	grain
h.	hour
H & P	history and physical
Hb; Hgb	hemoglobin
HBV	hepatitis B virus
HCT	hematocrit

Hgb	hemoglobin
HIV	human immunodeficiency virus (AIDS virus)
h/o	history of
HEENT	Head, ears, eyes, nose, throat
HT; HTN	hypertension
hx; Hx	history
I & O	intake and output
IBW	ideal body weight
ICP	intracranial pressure
ICU	intensive care unit
IDDM	insulin-dependent diabetes mellitus
IM	intramuscular; infectious mononucleosis
IV	intravenous
IVP	Intravenous push
K	potassium
kg	kilogram
KVO	keep vein open
L	left; liter; length; lumbar; lethal; pound
lat.	lateral
LLE	left lower extremity
LLL	left lower lobe
LLQ	left lower quadrant
LOC	level/loss of consciousness
LP	lumbar puncture
LR	lactated ringer's
LUE	left upper extremity
LUL	left upper lobe
LUQ	left upper quadrant
mg	milligram
mcg	microgram
mL	milliter
mm	millimeter, muscles
mmHg	millimeters of mercury
MRI	magnetic resonance imaging
MVA	motor vehicle accident

N/A	not applicable
Na	sodium
NaCl	sodium chloride
N & V; N/V	nausea and vomiting
NG; ng	nasogastic
NKA; NKDA	no known allergies; no known drug allergies
NPO; n.p.o.	nothing by mouth (*nil per os*)
NS	normal saline
NSAID	nonsteroidal anti-inflammatory drug
O	oxygen
O2	oxygen
OOB	out of bed
OR	operating room
OT	occupational therapy
OTC	over-the-counter
oz; Z	ounce
p	after
P-A; P/A; PA	posterior-anterior
P & A	percussion and auscultation
Pap test	Papanicolaou smear
PCA	patient-controlled analgesia
PERRLA	pupils equal, round, react to light and accommodation
PMH	past medical history
PMI	point of maximal impulse
PO; p.o.	orally (*per os*)
PPD	purified protein derivative (TB test)
PRN; p.r.n.	as required (*pro re nata*)
PSA	prostate-specific antigen
PT	prothrombin time; physical therapy
PTT	partial thromboplastin time
PVC	premature ventricular contraction
q.i.d.	four times daily (*quater in die*)
qd	once a day (*quaque die*)
℞	take
RBC; rbc	red blood cell; red blood count
RDA	recommended daily/dietary allowance

RDS	respiratory distress syndrome
RLE	right lower extremity
RLL	right lower lobe
RLQ	right lower quadrant
RML	right middle lobe of lung
R/O	rule out
ROM	range of motion
ROS	review of systems
RR	recovery room; respiratory rate
RT	radiation therapy; reading test; respiratory therapy
R/T	related to
RUE	right upper extremity
RUL	right upper lobe
RUQ	right upper quadrant
$\bar{s}$	without
SLE	systemic lupus erythematosus
SOB	shortness of breath
sol	solution dissolve
Sp.gr.; SG; s.g.	specific gravity
Staph	*Staphylococcus*
Stat	immediately (*statim*)
STD	sexually transmitted disease; skin test
Sub Q	subcutaneous injection
Strep	*Streptococcus*
s/s	signs & symptoms
Sx	symptoms
Sym	symmetrical
T	temperature
Tab	tablet
TAH	total abdominal hysterectomy
T & A	tonsillectomy and adenoidectomy
TB	tuberculin; tuberculosis; tubercle bacillus
t.i.d.	three times a day (*ter in die*)
TPN	total parenteral nutrition
TPR	temperature, pulse, respiration
TSE	testicular self-examination
TSH	thyroid-stimulating hormone

Tx	treatment
UA	urinalysis
UE	upper extremity
Umb; umb	umbilicus
URI	upper respiratory infection
US	ultrasound
UTI	urinary tract infection
UV	ultraviolet
vol	volume
V.S.; v.s.	vital signs
WBC; wbc	white blood cell; white blood count
WN	well nourished
WNL	within normal limits
wt	weight
y, yr	year
y/o	years old
Z; oz	ounce

Appendix B
Forming Plurals

The following chart contains information about the formation of plurals from the singular form. Use it to work on the frames that follow.

To Form Plurals	
If the singular ending is	The plural ending is
a	ae (pronounce ae as ī)
us	i
um	a
ma	mata
on	a
is	es
ix	ices } The word root is usually built from the plural forms of words ending in ix, ex, and ax (e.g., radix, radic/es, radic/otomy, radic/i/form).
ex	ices
ax	aces

bursae
bur′ sī
conjunctivae
kon junk′ tī vē
bacilli
bə sil′ ē

1.
Form the plural of

bursa ______________________

conjunctiva ______________________

bacillus ______________________

vertebra
ver′ tə bra
nucleus
nōō′ klē us
cornea
kor′ nē ə

2.
Give the singular form of

vertebrae ______________________

nuclei ______________________

corneas ______________________

atria ā′ trē ə cocci kok′ sē ilea (you pronounce) il′ ē ə	3. Form the plural of atrium ________ coccus ________ ileum ________
enema en′ ə mä bacterium ovum (you pronounce)	4. Give the singular form of enemata ________ bacteria ________ ova ________
cortices kor′ ti sēz fibromata fī brō′ mä tä protozoa prō′ to zō′ ə	5. Form the pleural of cortex ________ fibroma ________ protozoon ________
stigma stig′ mä prognosis prog nō′ sis spermatozoon sper mat′ ə zō ən	6. Give the singular form of stigmata ________ prognoses ________ spermatozoa ________
appendices (you pronounce) diagnoses dī ag nō′ sēz ganglia gang′ lē ä	7. Form the plural of appendix ________ diagnosis ________ ganglion ________
appendic	8. Refer to the table. Give the word root that usually refers to the appendix: ________.

cortic	the cortex ______________________
thorac (you pronounce)	the thorax ______________________
	9. With this new knowledge, which you found for yourself, build a word meaning
appendic/itis a pen di sī′ tis	inflammation of the appendix __________ / __________
cortic/al kor′ ti kəl	pertaining to the cortex __________ / __________
thorac/o/centesis thor′ ə kō sen tē′ sis	surgical puncture of the thorax __________ / _____ / __________
	10. Form the plural of
apices fornices varices sarcomata septa radii maxillae (you pronounce)	apex __________ fornex __________ varix __________ sarcoma __________ septum __________ radius __________ maxilla __________
	11. There are other ways of forming plurals. They apply to only a few words. When you meet these words and have a question about how their plural forms are built, consult a medical dictionary.

Appendix C
Medical Measurements

Volume		
Unit	**Abbreviation**	**Equivalency**
Liter	L	
Kiloliter	kl	1 kl = 1000 l
Milliliter	ml	1 L = 1000 ml
Cubic centimeter	cc	1 cc = 1 ml
Ounce	oz	1 oz = 30 ml
Dram	dr	1 dr = 4 ml
Drops	gtts	1 cc = 15 to 16 gtts*
Tablespoon	T	1 T = 15 ml
Teaspoon	t	1 t = 5 ml

Weight		
Unit	**Abbreviation**	**Equivalency**
Gram	g	
Kilogram	kg	1 kg = 1000 g
Milligram	mg	1 g = 1000 mg
Microgram	mcg	1 mg = 1000 mcg
Grain	gr	1 gr = 60 mg
Pound	lb	1 lb = 0.45 kg
Ounce	oz	1 oz = 28.35 g

Length		
Unit	**Abbreviation**	**Equivalency**
Meter	m	
Kilometer	kl	1 kl = 1000 m
Centimeter	cm	1 cm = 10 mm
Millimeter	mm	1 m = 1000 mm
Inch	in	1 in = 2.54 cm
Foot	ft	1 ft = 0.305 m

*Due to the different liquid surface tensions and specific gravity drop, conversions are approximations.

Index of Words and Word Parts

The following words and word parts are listed by page number.